MW00448470

The Happy Skin Solution

FIONA LAWSON

Copyright © 2019 Fiona Lawson

All rights reserved.

For my 16-year-old self, who longed for this book

CONTENTS

	Disclaimer	i
1	Acne, Science and You	Pg 1
2	Help Your Hormones	Pg 6
3	Look After Your Liver	Pg 16
4	Be Kind to Your Gut	Pg 26
5	Protect Your Skin's Barrier	Pg 38
6	Treat Yourself Well	Pg 46
7	Supplement Wisely	Pg 55
8	Make Happy Skin a Habit	Pg 63
	Appendix I	Pg 70
	Appendix II	Pg 72
	Appendix III	Pg 74

DISCLAIMER

The information contained in this book is intended to help readers make informed decisions about their health. It is designed to complement, not replace, medical treatment from a qualified healthcare practitioner. It should not be taken as a substitute for medical advice. If you have a medical problem, please see your doctor.

1. ACNE, SCIENCE AND YOU

Acne can take over your life.

It's not just that pimples can be a nuisance—it's how they make you feel about yourself. You're fearful of looking in the mirror every morning because of what might have emerged overnight. If your acne appears on your body as well as your face, you restrict what you wear and you dread warm weather. You've even been known to avoid social plans if you're having a bad skin day.

Your self-esteem crumbles with every new pimple. And, most frustrating of all, you feel as if you have no control over it.

The conventional approach to acne

It's easy to believe you're the only person suffering from this. But you're not. 'Acne vulgaris' (as it's medically known) affects up to 85% of adolescents and half of adults. It's the eighth most common affliction in the world, ahead of both asthma and back pain.

With so many people going through it, you'd think there'd be a solution. There are options—such as benzoyl peroxide gel, antibiotics and the potent drug isotretinoin (Roaccutane)—but they rarely work long-term. If you're one of the unlucky people whose acne resurged after a course of Roaccutane, you'll know that it comes back more stubbornly than ever.

You've tried facials, over-the-counter products and special supplements. You've experimented with your diet too. You may have cut out dairy or gluten or another 'trigger' food but—after weeks of boring meals and little improvement—you started eating normally again. Your GP or

1

dermatologist has told you diet doesn't affect acne anyway, so you keep looking for the next solution.

But what if I told you these 'solutions' are barely scratching the surface?

What acne is—and what it isn't

Let's be upfront: there's a lot we don't know about acne vulgaris. But what we do know is that it involves far more than your skin. Acne vulgaris is the exterior manifestation of a whole-body functioning issue that involves your hormones, gut, liver, immune system and more.

It may not feel like it, but a great deal has to happen for a spot to surface. Your body systems interact to create four key steps:

1) **Overproduction of facial oil.** This fatty substance, known as sebum, begins by blocking your pores.
2) **Abnormal skin cell shedding.** The skin cells in your pores stick together, further contributing to those blockages.
3) **Inflammation.** This immune response is what turns a simple blockage into a painful pimple. Inflammation can arise from too much sebum and too many skin cells but, confusingly, it can also cause too much sebum and too many skin cells.
4) **Microbial imbalance.** Too much of one type of skin bug (or not enough of another) can exacerbate the inflammatory response.

To further complicate matters, these steps overlap. And they're not even the start of the process, as an array of biochemical messages have to go awry before your body even gets to step one.

As you can see, a lot is going on. That's why we need to throw this pill-for-an-ill attitude out the window. Using one cream, taking one supplement or cutting out one food ('monotherapy') is not going to give you the clear complexion you crave. Your body is a brilliant, complex and dynamic entity—which means that it needs a multi-faceted approach to bring it back into balance.

Please don't mistake me: I'm not saying it's your fault that you have acne. Far from it. You've been dealt a genetic hand that you had no control over, and the way those genes are interacting with your environment (that is, all aspects of your life) has led to the development of acne. Someone can have the same diet and lifestyle as you but, because they have different genetic predispositions, their skin remains enviously clear.

Acne is an opportunity

The key to conquering your complexion is giving your body the tools it needs. Along with sleep, relaxation and appropriate exercise, one of the most powerful tools is food.

Food isn't just fuel for your body. It's information. We know that food influences our hormonal function, interacts with our immune system and shapes our gut microbiome (more on this later). The nutrients in food even interact with our genes.

Believe it or not, you can see acne as an opportunity. It's not happening to you—it's happening for you. By taking a whole-body approach to clearing your skin, you'll wind up making changes that positively impact your health as a whole. You'll learn how to nourish yourself inside and out.

This book will guide you through this approach so that it feels easy, relevant and actionable. But if you're still sceptical, I get it. It's important you know you can trust this advice. After all, haven't you already tried so much?

Before we delve into what you can do, let's take a moment to chat about the evidence surrounding food and acne—its value, its limitations, and how you can use it to make your own decisions.

What can you believe?

'Evidence-based' is the buzzword in healthcare these days, and for good reason. With the rise of social media, it seems anyone can give health advice. It's up to you, as the consumer of this advice, to work out who you can trust—and it's not always an easy task.

But have you ever stopped to think about what 'evidence-based' means? Most people presume it means a product has been tested in a scientific trial, but it's not quite that simple. The notion of 'evidence' is far from black-and-white.

What is evidence?

Let's take a quick look at how evidence is generated, and why we run into problems when studying food and health.

In a 'gold-standard' trial, one randomly assigned group of people receives the product, and another randomly assigned group receives a placebo (a sugar pill). Neither the people giving the product nor the people receiving it know if it's the real one or the placebo to reduce the risk of bias. After a set time period, differences are observed or measured between the two groups. If the group receiving the product has improved more than the group receiving the placebo, then the product is deemed to be effective.

You're probably wondering what all this has to do with food and acne. Well, quite a lot. As you can see, the gold-standard trial works very well when you're testing a drug. In this instance, you're changing one thing and waiting to see if it has one, specific result.

Food doesn't work like that. Unlike drugs, food affects lots of body systems at once. Whereas drugs are designed to work quickly, the effect of food is also slow and cumulative. If you truly wanted to test the impact of one food on acne, you'd have to hold a clinical trial for *years*. You'd also have to control everything that people eat! Sadly, this sort of trial isn't realistic.

Instead, most of what we know about nutrition and its effect on health comes from epidemiological studies. That's just a clever way of saying, 'Observe a group of people over a set time period and see if any patterns emerge.' This can be illuminating but—because you can't control all the influencing factors like you can in a gold-standard trial—you have to be more cautious about the results.

The bottom line? Nutrition is hard to study, which means there are huge holes in what scientists have researched.

Evidence and acne

When your doctor or dermatologist says food doesn't affect acne, they're abiding by their regulations. It's true that there's little high-quality research confirming the impact of food on acne (or otherwise) and medical practitioners have to reflect this.

But that doesn't mean food doesn't impact acne. To illustrate this, let's consider smoking and lung cancer. Until a seminal study observed 40,000 cigarette-smoking doctors in the 1960s, we had no evidence that smoking caused lung cancer. Researchers followed the doctors for ten years and found that the more they smoked, the more likely they were to a) get lung cancer and b) die.

This trial wasn't even gold-standard, and yet the data was so strong that scientists took it as proof that smoking causes lung cancer. But does that mean that smoking wasn't causing lung cancer before—simply because a scientific study hadn't taken place to prove it? I'll leave you to decide.

Evidence is personal

I'm not suggesting we throw all evidence out the window. I wholeheartedly believe in the value of well-designed human studies, but they're only one part of the picture. If we want to help ourselves, it's also important we pay attention to the two other principles of evidence-based medicine:

1) Clinical judgement

2) Patient's values and preferences

That means that along with studies and trials, you can draw from a qualified practitioner's experience of what's worked with other people *and* your wishes. That last bit is important. You should honour your instincts, as no one else is ever going to know what it's like to live in your body.

This book aims to channel all three principles of the evidence-based approach to help you achieve clear, glowing skin. You'll uncover the foods and habits that can help to conquer acne. You'll discover how changing your thoughts can positively influence your complexion. You'll find out which supplements can help you, and how to take them.

Most of all, you'll free yourself from constantly worrying about your skin.

How to use this book

My experience of working with clients has shown me that some people love to know the 'why' behind recommendations—while others just want to know what to do.

You can use this book either way. If you want all the juicy detail, read each chapter all the way through. If you want a quick summary and action points, skip to the 'Quick Read' and 'Take Action' sections at the start and end of each chapter.

In the journey to clear skin we'll go through your hormones, gut, liver, acid mantle and mind. Everyone's acne is different, but I'll help you work out where you need to pay the most attention.

Are you ready to love your skin? Let's begin.

2. HELP YOUR HORMONES

Remember: acne involves several body systems. Pay close attention to this chapter if:
- *You feel nauseous on rising*
- *You crave sweet foods*
- *You have mood swings*
- *You have lots of phlegm and/or mucous*
- *You have a history of childhood ear infections*
- *You have dry skin*
- *Your body mass index is more than 25*

QUICK READ
- Your skin type is influenced by your genetics, your environment and your hormones.
- Hormonal function plays a key role in sebum production and inflammation, both of which drive acne.
- You can help to balance your hormones by regulating your blood sugar, eating the right fats and determining the right amount of dairy for you.

You've likely been told that acne is caused by oily skin. This is true—but it's only one chapter in the story. Have you ever stopped to wonder why your skin is 'too oily' in the first place? And how does this oiliness lead to inflammatory acne?

Far from being fixed, your skin type is adaptable. It's shaped by your genetics, your environment and your hormones. The first one you can't do anything about, and the second one—which in this case is the temperature and the humidity—is largely out of your control too. But you can do a lot to influence the third one: your hormones.

An easy way to understand hormones is to think of them as little chemical messengers. Your body is constantly looking for signals from your internal and external worlds and, once it interprets those signals, it releases hormones to tell your cells what to do. Consider sleep: when your body senses it's getting dark outside, it releases the hormone melatonin to help you wind down.

A major signal that directs hormones is the food we eat. And to help the hormones that impact acne, we need to focus on three areas:

1) Balancing blood sugar
2) Being mindful about dairy
3) Eating the right fats

Let's take a look at each in detail.

1) <u>Help your hormones by…Balancing blood sugar</u>

Here's an area in which the research is encouraging: one study found that after ten weeks of eating a diet that balances blood sugar, patients not only saw improvements in their acne, but their sebum-producing glands also shrunk. Another study found that eating a blood-sugar-balancing diet changed patients' sebum composition and reduced their number of pimples.

To understand why this happens, we need to take a quick look at a master hormone: insulin.

Every time you eat, your pancreas releases insulin. This helps to get the sugar (glucose) out of your bloodstream and into your cells, so that they have the energy to carry out their important functions.

Insulin is essential—but we can run into problems when too much is released too often. This is because excess insulin increases the production of androgens, a group of hormones which includes testosterone. Testosterone kicks your sebaceous glands into overdrive, which winds up making your skin more oily and more acne-prone.

Put more simply:

more insulin → more androgens → more testosterone → more oil → more pimples.

Since its main job is to shuttle glucose around, insulin is most spiked by foods that:

a) contain high levels of glucose
b) are digested rapidly

In essence, this means anything white, fluffy or sweet. When it comes to clear skin, sugar and simple carbohydrates are not your friends.

Does this seem like old news to you? If so, great. Knowledge is the first step. The second step is understanding how to put that knowledge into action. Here's what to do:

a) Cut down on sugar

Let's start with the good news: conquering acne does not mean you have to swear off dessert forever. But, while you're making a concerted effort to help your skin recalibrate, it makes sense to cut down on insulin-spiking sugar.

Some sources of sugar are obvious, such as cakes, sweets, biscuits, honey and jam. But some are more subtle: cereals, condiments (including ketchup) and ready-made sauces are surprisingly high in the sweet stuff. Get into the habit of checking ingredients labels—if a product has more than 5g of sugar per 100g, it's best to choose something else.

Fruit is the exception to this. While it can be high in sugar, it's also rich in fibre and phytonutrients (more on these in chapter 3), which means it's a valuable part of a skin-supporting diet. Good choices include berries, apples, plums and pears. While your skin is calming down, it's best not to have extra-sweet varieties more than a couple of times a week. These include grapes, pineapple, mango and bananas.

The only category of sweet things that I would recommend cutting out entirely is sugary drinks—so avoid both fizzy drinks and fruit juices. These contain a hefty dose of sugar that shoots straight into your bloodstream. Your skin and your health as a whole will be much better off without them.

b) Make clever swaps

The second tactic for balancing your blood sugar is to replace simple carbohydrates with complex ones. Complex carbohydrates are higher in fibre, which means they're digested more slowly and therefore help to maintain a skin-friendly level of insulin.

Give your skin a break by making the following swaps:

Food	Clever swap
White bread	Wholegrain, rye or spelt bread
White rice	Brown, red or wild rice

White pasta	Wholegrain or brown rice pasta
Cereal	Porridge oats
Couscous	Quinoa

Be your own health detective. Many 'brown' loaves of bread are still made with white flour, so it pays to read ingredients labels.

You might be wondering why I don't recommend swapping potatoes for something else. White potatoes have received a bad rap in recent years but, if eaten with a dose of common sense, they certainly have a place on a skin-supporting diet. Highly processed chips and crisps are out, but gently boiled or baked potatoes are in—especially if you eat them in line with the next point.

c) Create a smart plate

The final tactic for achieving even blood sugar is to slow digestion.

Every time you eat carbohydrate (complex or otherwise), pair it with a form of protein and/or healthy fat. Protein and fat take much longer for your body to digest, which means they slow the release of glucose into your bloodstream. If you're not sure which foods fall into which categories, check the lists in Appendix I.

Just to recap: a slower release of glucose means a smaller spike in insulin. A smaller spike in insulin means less sebum. Less sebum means fewer blemishes.

Eating for slow digestion is easy when you get into the habit. If you're reaching for an apple (complex carbohydrate), simply pair it with a handful of nuts (protein and fat). Craving that baked potato (complex carbohydrate)? Serve it with a succulent fillet of cod (protein) with a drizzle of olive oil (fat).

Balancing blood sugar is such a crucial step for conquering acne that it's worth going over again. We can sum it up in three simple points:

a) Minimise your sugar intake
b) Favour complex carbohydrates
c) Eat protein and/or healthy fat with every meal or snack

As well as regulating sebum production, you'll also notice this way of eating steadies your appetite. You can expect side effects of greater energy and renewed focus.

2) Help your hormones by…Being mindful about dairy

Dairy causes acne, right? You may be surprised to learn that, well, it depends.

The research in this area is far from conclusive. As part of the Nurses' Health Study II, researchers asked 47,355 women what they ate as teenagers and whether they had acne. Based on their responses, it was determined that the more milk they drank, the more likely they were to have acne as a teen.

But, as with any research, we need to apply critical thinking to the results. There are two issues with this sort of study:

1) People are notoriously unreliable when remembering what they ate. Can you recall what you had for breakfast a week ago, let alone 20 years ago?
2) Correlation does not equal causation. The increased rate of acne in milk-drinkers could be down to chance, or down to something else entirely. You may notice that the sun has risen when you wake up— but that doesn't mean your waking-up is making the sun rise!

And yet the dairy-acne connection is corroborated elsewhere. Another piece of research—a review of several studies—found that people who consumed dairy were 25% more likely to suffer from acne. If they drank more than two glasses of milk per day, there were 43% more likely to have acne.

How dairy stokes the acne fire

The research and my clinical experience lead me to believe that dairy does worsen acne *in some people*. Let's look at why:

1) **Casein sensitivity**. If you're sensitive to A1 beta-casein, a protein in cow's dairy, it can cause an inflammatory reaction that shows up on your complexion. These are the people who have dramatic results when they cut out cow's dairy. They also find that eating some goat's and/or sheep's dairy is fine because these contain a different form of beta-casein.
2) **Whey sensitivity**. This is another type of protein found in cow's milk. Like casein, it can cause problems in some people. It also increases insulin. Together, these contribute to the 'bodybuilder acne' that can develop when people eat lots of whey-based protein powder.

3) **Hormonal interplay**. This is how dairy affects the rest of us. You've likely heard that milk contains hormones—and the theory is that they mess with your hormones and give you those breakouts. But the interplay between acne and dairy is far more complex than this.

Dairy and hormones

Dairy does contain some hormones, but its impact on acne likely stems from the messages it's giving our bodies. Remember, food is information.

Studies show that drinking milk causes our liver to create more of a hormone called insulin-like growth factor-1 (or IGF-1 for short). As the name suggests, IGF-1 gives cells in the body the message that it's time to start growth processes. Emerging research shows there are other substances in milk, called microRNAs, which are also designed to encourage cell proliferation. In this way, milk is not just food—it's software. Milk programmes offspring to grow.

Cow's milk is designed to help a calf double its birth weight in 40 days. It may be that these growth signals are too much for an adult human. When a person no longer needs to grow, the signals start misfiring—instructing skin cells to multiply too quickly, and causing sebaceous glands to produce too much oil. Together, these block pores and lead to pimples.

One study found that levels of IGF-1 in women's blood correlated with the severity of their acne. So, if you know that dairy raises IGF-1, is it worth cutting back?

What to do about dairy

The reason I've talked you through all the above is so you can see how nuanced this topic is. It's not as simple as dairy = acne. The key is to find out how *you* react to dairy.

For three months, I recommend cutting out all forms of dairy. This includes milk, cream, yoghurt, ice cream, cheese and butter.

After three months, begin the process of reintroduction, in this order:

1) Butter
2) Fermented milk (kefir)
3) Hard cheese: Parmesan, Grana Padano, mature cheddar
4) Yoghurt
5) Soft cheese: cream cheese, Brie
6) Cream
7) Milk
8) Ice cream

Eat the food three times in one day (i.e. three servings of butter), then wait three days. If your skin doesn't react, you can eat that food once more. If your skin does react, continue to eliminate it and move to the next type of dairy on the list.

For those types of dairy that you did react to, try eating a sheep or goat's milk alternative and see if it makes a difference.

In my experience, most people who've suffered from acne should avoid making dairy a mainstay of their diet. But they can find a happy equilibrium. Your skin may be fine with hard cheese, but not great after a latte. One serving of dairy a day could be OK, but you start to see issues after two.

Experiment and see what works for you. The goal is to make your diet as diverse and relaxed as possible.

3) Help your hormones by…Eating the right fats

Poor old fat was shunned for decades. From heart disease to obesity, it was the scapegoat for countless conditions—and we embraced low-fat eating as a result.

Avocados were out, but low-fat cookies were in. Egg whites stayed in vogue, but egg yolks were washed down the sink. Butter nearly disappeared from our shelves due to fat phobia.

Thankfully, things are turning around for fat. We now realise that a healthy amount of fat is vital for our health, and that includes happy hormones and glowing skin. Fats influence hormonal function in lots of ways, including:

- Providing **raw material** for hormone production. That's right, some of your hormones are *made* from fat.
- Creating strong and **flexible** cell membranes. These enable hormones to dock onto receptors and deliver their message effectively.
- Making **prostaglandins**. Some fats are turned into prostaglandins—hormone-like substances that regulate inflammation.

So, eating healthy fats helps to balance hormones and calm skin. But, like with anything in nutrition, there are many sides to the story. Let's take a look at the different types of fats and how they influence acne specifically.

Saturated fats
Predominantly in: butter, coconut oil, meat, dairy

We do need some saturated fat, but too much can aggravate acne because it increases IGF-1 and activates those growth pathways. It can also change the composition of sebum and make it more inflammatory.

Some of these effects may be reduced by eating saturated fat with a hefty dose of fibre. You'll learn more about the value of fibre in chapter 4.

Monounsaturated fats
Predominantly in: olive oil, avocados, olives, nuts, seeds

Monounsaturated fat is beneficial for hormonal health and it has anti-inflammatory action, both of which have a knock-on effect on acne.

Eat this type of fat daily, but don't put it *on* your face. As you'll discover in chapter 5, using monounsaturated fats in your skincare routine can make acne worse.

Polyunsaturated fats
Omega-3 fats predominantly in: oily fish, chia seeds, flaxseeds
Omega-6 fats predominantly in: nuts, seeds, vegetable oils

Your body can make other types of fats, but it can't make omega-3 and omega-6 polyunsaturated fats—so you need to get them from your diet.

But the balance of these fats is important. For millennia humans ate omega-6 and omega-3 in a ratio of 3:1 (perhaps even 1:1) but, thanks to the rise of processed food, we're now more likely to eat them in a ratio of 16:1.

This is a problem. Omega-6 fats get turned into pro-inflammatory prostaglandins (those hormone-like substances) in the body, while omega-3 fats get turned into anti-inflammatory prostaglandins. If your pro-inflammatory prostaglandins outnumber your anti-inflammatory ones, it increases the severity of inflammatory processes i.e. acne.

Thankfully, it also goes the other way. A study of 1,000 teenagers found that those who ate more omega-3 rich seafood enjoyed fewer symptoms of acne.

Trans/hydrogenated fats
Predominantly in: margarine, fast food, shop-bought baked goods

This a synthetic form of fat that was designed to be shelf-stable. Your body doesn't like it. This type of fat is best avoided altogether.

Make the most of fat

You'll have noticed a theme when it comes to fats: inflammation. Eating the right fats is just one part of the much bigger picture of decreasing the inflammatory load on your body, which is ultimately what this book is about.

And yet, like dairy, it pays to be mindful about fats—but not obsessive. After all, all foods that contain fat have several types of fat together. Take mackerel: it's known for its omega-3 content, but most people are surprised to discover that it also contains more saturated fat than a fillet steak!

Your skin seeks balance. With that in mind, here are some fat-eating principles to follow:

- Use **saturated fats** (such as coconut oil and butter) for high-heat cooking, as they remain stable at high temperatures. Be mindful of consuming too many saturated fats otherwise.
- Enjoy a serving of **monounsaturated fat or polyunsaturated fat** with each meal. This could be a tablespoon of olive oil, a quarter of an avocado or a sprinkle of seeds. Get creative.
- Eat oily fish two to three times per week. If you're a vegan or vegetarian, eat chia seeds or flaxseeds three to four times per week. These are all valuable sources of anti-inflammatory **omega-3** fats.
- Don't shy away from sensible portions of nuts and seeds, but avoid processed seed/vegetable oils such as sunflower oil, corn oil and soybean oil. These make it easy to overconsume **omega-6** fats.
- Avoid all sources of **trans fats**.

Well done!

With balanced blood sugar, healthy fat intake and a personalised approach to dairy, you've already taken a huge step to regulating sebum production, reducing inflammation and clearing your skin.

There's more to discover. In the next chapter, you'll learn what your acne has to do with your liver—and how you can eat to support healthy detoxification.

TAKE ACTION

Here's a recap of what to do:

- ✓ Cut down on sugar. Check ingredients labels—if something has more than 5g sugar per 100g, reconsider eating it. Fruit is an exception to this.

- ✓ Replace simple carbohydrates (white bread, pasta and rice) with complex carbohydrates. Good choices include rye bread, wild rice, wholegrain pasta, oats and quinoa.

- ✓ Eat a source of protein and/or healthy fat with every meal and snack.

- ✓ Eliminate dairy for three months. Then, reintroduce it by testing one form at a time. You'll likely find that your skin can tolerate some dairy.

- ✓ Use saturated fats for high-heat cooking, and enjoy monounsaturated and polyunsaturated fats (such as olive oil and avocado) with your meals.

- ✓ Enjoy oily fish or chia seeds/flaxseeds a few times a week. Eat sensible portions of nuts and seeds, and try to avoid vegetable oils and seed oils.

- ✓ Avoid all sources of trans fat, including margarine and fast food.

3. LOOK AFTER YOUR LIVER

Pay close attention if, along with acne, you experience:
- *Headaches*
- *Night sweats*
- *Chemical or odour sensitivities*
- *Chronic itching*
- *Fatigue and/or sluggishness*
- *PMS*

QUICK NOTES
- You come into contact with thousands of toxins every day. Your liver has to deal with them all.
- If there's a mismatch between your toxic load and your liver's ability to detoxify it, this can lead to hormonal imbalance that worsens acne.
- You can promote clear skin by both maximising your detoxification function and minimising your exposure to toxins.

What do you think when you hear the word, 'detox'? For many, it conjures images of juice fasts, superfood powders and raw-food meals. It's easy to dismiss the concept as marketing hype.

But detoxification is a fundamental physiological function—and it has a tremendous impact on your skin. And, contrary to what marketers would have you believe, you don't support detoxification by eating less. You support it by eating *more* of the right things.

Detoxification 101

Your body has to process hundreds of chemicals as you go about your daily business. These include the obvious sources—such as pollution in the air and pesticides on food—but there are also less-obvious sources that contribute to the load.

You may be surprised to learn that you ingest microscopic amounts of the following:

- **Plastics** from food containers
- **Chemicals** from cosmetics and cleaning products
- **Fire retardant sprays** from sofas and clothes
- **Teflon** from cookware and bakeware
- **Volatile organic compounds** from paint
- **Additives** from food
- **Dust, bacteria and moulds** from indoor air
- **Chemicals** from drinking water
- **Heavy metals** from pollution

These are just a few examples. While it's true that individual products contain safe amounts of the various toxins, nobody really knows what happens when they accumulate over several years. Again, this is an area in which a long-term trial would be neither feasible nor ethical. And yet you could argue we're all part of a long-term trial—simply because we're exposed to more chemicals than ever before.

What this means is that your liver is working hard. As your major organ of detoxification, it's continually breaking down substances and repackaging them up so they can be safely shuttled out of the body. This process is known as 'biotransformation'.

Detoxification and acne

A popular theory is that your liver is so 'congested' with these toxins that it ends up pushing some of them out via your skin. Although your skin is an organ of elimination, there's no evidence that this seeping of toxins is behind acne. In fact, studies show that 95% to 99% of acne sufferers have normal liver function.

And yet, when you support the liver, acne improves. So, what's happening?

It's more likely that there's a mismatch between the detoxification load and the nutrients required to handle that load effectively. This means that some of the liver's less critical functions—such as eliminating used hormones and other by-products of metabolism—are compromised.

If you're not eliminating hormones, you'll have higher levels of them. High levels of testosterone (a type of androgen hormone found in both men and women) can be problematic in those of us prone to acne because our skin more readily converts it into dihydrotestosterone (DHT). Stick with me here!

DHT is even more potent than testosterone. It's like Jekyll and Hyde: Jekyll (testosterone) carries out important work but, when he turns into Hyde (DHT), he goes on the rampage. DHT uses its Hyde-like strength to encourage the sebaceous glands to produce more oil and, as you learnt in chapter 2, more oil often means more blemishes.

And that's just the recirculating hormones. Like a factory producing smoke, every cell of your body is producing waste products all the time. Your liver has to deal with all of those too.

So, let's pull this together:

high toxic load + not enough nutrients = an overloaded liver.

An overloaded liver → higher levels of used hormones and metabolic waste products in the body → more inflammation and more sebum → acne.

As you can see, it's not so much the 'seeping' of toxins that contributes to acne, but the fact that a high toxic load creates other acne-driving imbalances.

But what about acne sufferers having those normal liver enzymes? Well, there's a spectrum. There's a big difference between a liver that's functioning within a 'normal' range and a liver that's functioning optimally. For clear skin, you want your liver operating at its best.

The good news is there are two ways to support your liver's biotransformation:

1) Maximise your detoxification function.
2) Minimise your exposure to toxins.

In this chapter, I'll show you how to do both.

How to maximise your detoxification function

Way back in the 1950s, researchers in Japan found that you could improve acne through supporting the liver with targeted nutrients.

The concept was pioneering at the time, but now there are thousands of studies showing that certain foods can boost liver function. This is because they contain the amino acids, vitamins and minerals that the liver needs to carry out its stages of biotransformation. Plant foods also contain phytonutrients—special substances that act as a further buffer to the damage caused by toxins as they're broken down.

By selecting these functional foods, you're giving your detoxification a gentle nudge. The gentle part is important: this form of detoxification support is designed to be both safe and sustainable.

For a happy liver and healthy skin, here's what you should be eating more of:

Protein Your liver takes the amino acids from protein and attaches them to toxins. This makes the toxins water-soluble, so you can get them out of your body more easily. Get into the habit of eating high-quality protein with every meal. Good choices include eggs, chicken, fish, seafood, nuts, pulses and legumes.
Serving: the size of your palm

Crucifers This liver-loving family of vegetables include broccoli, cauliflower, kale, watercress, rocket, cabbage, turnips, Brussels sprouts, radish, pak choi and spring greens. They contain special phytonutrients that upregulate enzymes in your liver, enabling them to deal with used hormones more effectively.
Serving: 1 heaped handful (when cooked)

Berries The process of breaking down toxins can lead to the release of skin-damaging free radicals. Dark-coloured berries are rich in the antioxidants required to neutralise those free radicals. Go for blackcurrants, redcurrants, raspberries, blueberries, strawberries and blackberries. Fresh or frozen is fine.
Serving: 1 heaped handful

Garlic Have you ever noticed that garlic becomes sticky when you chop it? That stickiness comes from special compounds which attach themselves to toxins, helping you to get them out of your body. Try to eat some garlic every day.
Serving: 1 clove

Grapefruit The ability of this fruit to influence liver function is well-known—so much so that people taking statins and antihistamines have to be wary of it, as it affects the activity of drug-metabolising enzymes in the

liver. But it's that ability to tinker with enzymes that makes it helpful at regulating your toxic load. (If you're on medication, check with your doctor before eating grapefruit.)
Serving: ½ grapefruit

Beetroot This is rich in folate and phytonutrients, both of which are required to break down toxins. Beetroot is especially good for acne sufferers as it has anti-inflammatory qualities too. If you buy pre-cooked beetroot, look for one without added sugar.
Serving: 2 medium beetroot

Green tea This antioxidant-rich drink can improve liver enzyme levels and reduce levels of DHT. Aim for three cups a day, but avoid drinking it on an empty stomach (as it can make you feel nauseous).
Serving: 1 cup

Turmeric This vibrant spice not only helps liver enzymes, but it also encourages bile production. Bile gets your digestive system going—helping you to excrete metabolised toxins (a.k.a. do a poo!). Eat turmeric with black pepper and a little healthy fat to enhance its effectiveness.
Serving: 1 teaspoon

Extra virgin olive oil This is rich in antioxidants (helping to fight those free radicals) and, like turmeric, it can stimulate bile production. The best extra virgin olive oil comes from a single origin rather than a blend.
Serving: 1 tablespoon

Lemon Limonene, a phytonutrient in lemon rind, supports your detoxification pathways and gets your digestive juices flowing. Squeeze the juice of half a lemon (preferably organic and unwaxed) into a mug of hot water, and pop the rind into the cup!
Serving: ½ lemon

Herbs Coriander is a natural 'chelator', which means it binds to heavy metals. Other common herbs—such as parsley, rosemary and mint—have liver-supporting properties too. Sprinkle fresh herbs over salads, or use dried herbs in soups and casseroles.
Serving: 1 handful fresh or 1 tablespoon dried

Flaxseed This increases a special hormone-binding substance in your body, thus reducing the load on your liver. It's also a vegetarian source of omega-3 fats. If possible, grind flaxseed just before you eat it.
Serving: 1 tablespoon ground flaxseed

Water Not a food, but certainly worth mentioning. Water makes all biochemical reactions within cells possible, including those involved in biotransformation. To make water more interesting, infuse it with fresh fruit or herbs.
Serving: a minimum of 8 glasses or 2 litres each day

Aim to eat at least three liver-supporting foods daily. It needn't be difficult: pair scrambled eggs on toast with a rocket side salad and a drizzle of olive oil, and you've already hit your three foods. Enjoy a cup of green tea with some berries for dessert, and you've bumped it up to five.

A common feature of nutritional therapy is that the sum is greater than the parts, and that's especially true here. That handful of rocket may seem insignificant—but consistently eating to support your liver can make a huge difference over time.

How to minimise your exposure to toxins

Boosting detoxification is just one side of the coin. Your skin will also thank you if you lighten the load on your liver.

As you've learnt, we come into contact with hundreds of toxins every day. We can't avoid them all—but we can take steps to minimise our exposure. Start here:

- If you **smoke** or take recreational drugs, stop. A single burning cigarette releases 7,000 chemicals. I appreciate it can be hard to kick the habit, but it's essential for both your skin and your health as a whole. Many people find hypnotherapy helpful here.
- Try not to run or walk by **busy roads**—choose another route.
- Cut down on **plastic**. Get a stainless steel water bottle, invest in glass storage containers for the fridge and use baking parchment instead of cling film. Never use plastic in the microwave.
- Gradually **replace your non-stick cookware**. Glass baking dishes and ceramic pans are good alternatives.
- Switch your **skincare and body-care products** to organic versions. This is more important for anything that you leave on (such as moisturiser) over anything you rinse off (such as shower gel).
- Reconsider your use of **perfume or aftershave**. Rather than wearing it every day, save it for special occasions or use natural

fragrance instead. Orange blossom essential oil (diluted in a carrier oil) can be an uplifting option.

- **Dry clean** your clothes as little as possible. For gentle cleaning, consider using a cool cycle in your washing machine instead.
- Pay attention to your **oral hygiene** by brushing and flossing twice a day. Visit the hygienist at least once a year.
- Choose **organic food** as much as you can within the realms of your budget. Prioritise buying organic food in this order: meat, eggs and dairy, fruits and vegetables. Organic or not, wash all fruits and vegetables before eating.
- **Cook from scratch** as much as you can, as this will naturally reduce your intake of food additives. Favour recipes that use minimal processed and packaged foods, including canned goods.
- **Filter your tap water**. You can install a water filter in your home or simply use a freestanding filter jug.
- Take steps to **clean the air** in your home. You may wish to:
  a) Buy a few snake plants and spider plants to go in your most-used rooms.
  b) Get rid of synthetic diffusers and use natural potpourri instead.
  c) If redecorating, choose paints that are labelled no-VOC or low-VOC.
  d) Swap your cleaning products for environmentally friendly brands. Spirit vinegar and bicarbonate of soda can be used as multi-purpose cleaning products too.
- Investigate your home for **damp or mould**. This is particularly relevant if your acne started shortly after you moved to a new house. If you do find mould, you may need to engage a professional to get rid of it.

Reading this list can be scary. Suddenly it seems there are potential skin hazards everywhere! While it pays to be mindful about this, it's not worth getting stressed over (especially because—as you'll learn in chapter 6—the stress can be even worse for your skin).

Begin by making small changes. Today, recycle your plastic water bottle and treat yourself to that stainless steel one you've been eyeing up. Tomorrow, floss your teeth in the evening. The next day, choose organic eggs in the supermarket.

Yet again, the sum is greater than the parts. Little changes soon add up to a big reduction in your toxic load.

Food and the biotransformation burden

Just as there are foods that support biotransformation, there are some that can scupper it. While you're working to clear your skin, it's also worth paying close attention to the following:

Alcohol

Your body views alcohol as a toxin. As soon as it's ingested, getting rid of it becomes your liver's number one priority—meaning other substances aren't detoxified as efficiently. Not only this, but alcohol also depletes your body's store of B vitamins and the master antioxidant glutathione, both of which are essential for healthy skin.

I'm not saying you should never have a drink again—no one wants to be the person refusing champagne at a party! But, for the sake of your skin, save it for special occasions.

Caffeine

Too much caffeine can increase stress hormones and disrupt blood sugar, driving the inflammation behind acne.

But 'too much' is different for everyone. Some people have liver enzymes that metabolise caffeine in as little as five hours, while others take up to 11. If you feel jittery, anxious or have difficulty sleeping, it's likely you're consuming too much for you.

Experiment and find your balance. To reduce the load on your liver and to further help your hormones, it's best to drink caffeinated drinks such as coffee and tea (including green tea) in the morning and only after food.

Large fish

Hang on, isn't fish good for you? It is—but the trouble is so many fish live in polluted waters. This pollution, which includes the heavy metal mercury, gets into their food supply and accumulates in their tissues.

You then enjoy a fillet of tuna, and get a dose of mercury that your liver has to deal with. It isn't surprising that research has found a correlation between exposure to heavy metals and fatty liver disease.

Larger fish accumulate more heavy metals, which is why it's a good idea to limit your intake of tuna, marlin, swordfish, king mackerel and shark. One portion of these fish each week is plenty.

Another one down!

Let's recap: you've balanced your blood sugar, boosted your healthy fat intake and addressed dairy. Now you're supporting your liver and dialling down your toxic load.

With each step, you're taking away the fuel for acne's fire. And there's so much more we can do. Next up: how to optimise your digestion and gut bacteria to further clear your skin.

TAKE ACTION

Here's a recap of what to do:

✓ Eat high-quality protein with every meal or snack (you'll already be doing this if you've read chapter 1!). Your liver especially likes eggs, chicken, fish and seafood.

✓ Eat at least three servings of liver-supporting foods daily. These include:
  - Cruciferous vegetables
  - Berries
  - Garlic
  - Grapefruit
  - Beetroot
  - Green tea
  - Turmeric
  - Extra virgin olive oil
  - Lemon
  - Herbs

Flick back to earlier in the chapter to see what constitutes a serving for each.

✓ If you smoke, find the help you need to stop.

✓ Take small steps to reduce your exposure to toxins. You can:
  - Swap plastic food containers for glass versions
  - Replace your non-stick cookware with ceramic pans
  - Switch your skincare to organic versions
  - Stop wearing perfume every day
  - Choose organic food as much as you can
  - Cook from scratch
  - Filter your tap water
  - Fill your home with plants
  - Swap your cleaning products for environmentally friendly versions

✓ Save drinking alcohol for special occasions.

✓ Drink caffeinated drinks only after eating food. If you're drinking the right amount of caffeine for you, you should feel alert but not jittery.

✓ Avoid eating large fish (including tuna) more than once a week.

4. BE KIND TO YOUR GUT

Pay close attention if, along with acne, one of more the following apply to you:
- *You barely have time to think about what you're eating*
- *You feel bloated soon after eating*
- *Your toilet habits are unpredictable*
- *You've taken one or more courses of antibiotics in your life*
- *You frequently get ill*
- *You often feel fatigued*

QUICK READ
- Although we can't yet explain all the mechanisms, we know that your gut and your skin are inherently linked.
- People who suffer from acne are more likely to have low stomach acid, bacterial overgrowth and/or microbiome disruption.
- You can promote clear skin by looking after your gut. This involves addressing both what and how you eat.

Our obsession with gut health may seem new, but did you know that we've been aware of a connection between the gut and the skin for almost a century?

In 1930, two pioneering dermatologists, John Stokes and Donald Pillsbury, suggested that emotional states could alter the gut microbiome. They believed this could lead to leaky gut and inflammation—contributing to skin conditions such as acne.

It turns out they were onto something. The 'gut-skin axis' is a new and exciting area of research, and one which is adding further weight to the idea that the gut and its microbiome has a dramatic impact on other parts of the body.

We'll discuss the gut microbiome in detail below. For now, consider these three points:

1) There are lots of **similarities between your gut and your skin**. Both tissues have a rich blood supply, both act as interfaces between the body and the outside world, and both are home to diverse communities of bacteria.
2) It's well accepted that **some gut conditions can have skin manifestations**. Chronic blisters can be a symptom of Coeliac disease. People with Crohn's disease are more likely to develop psoriasis.
3) You need **food to supply the nutrients that maintain your skin's health**. If you're not breaking down food effectively—a.k.a. if your gut is struggling—your skin can suffer.

In the absence of a robust randomised, controlled trial, is it too much to wonder if compromised gut health contributes to acne?

I'll leave you to form your own opinion. In this chapter, we'll visit every stage of digestion. We'll look at why problems arise, how this may affect your skin, and what you can do about it.

As we go through, think about your digestion and eating habits. One of these points may spark a light-bulb moment.

The mouth

What happens:
Your mouth is where digestion begins. Not only do you chew to physically break down food, but enzymes in your saliva also get to work to begin the chemical breakdown.

What can go wrong:
Not many of us chew well. If we're not eating in a rush, we're distracted by something else. Have you ever got through an entire meal and realised you didn't taste any of it?

The nub of the issue is very simple here: if you don't chew well, you send larger bits of food down into your stomach and small intestine. This puts stress on your digestive system and means you don't absorb as many skin-supporting nutrients from your food.

What to do:

Don't worry, I'm not going to tell you to chew every mouthful 20 times! In my experience, that's rarely an effective long-term strategy. But here's what I do recommend:

a) Only eat when sitting down. This is a simple tactic to bring more focus to your food.
b) Put your knife and fork down between each mouthful. This automatically slows you down.

Proper chewing is powerful. For some people, it's all they need to dramatically improve their digestion, which has a knock-on effect on their skin.

The stomach

What happens:

After you swallow, your food travels down your oesophagus to your stomach. Here it's submerged in stomach acid to kill off any bacteria, and churned to further break it down. The enzyme pepsin digests protein here too.

What can go wrong:

You're probably familiar with the concept of having too much stomach acid. After all, that's what all those over-the-counter heartburn pills are for.

But opinion is shifting on this, and it's now believed that in some people those symptoms are down to *low* stomach acid. Stokes and Pillsbury were ahead of their time here too—they hypothesised that up to 40% of people with acne have low stomach acid.

Without sufficient acid to kill off bacteria, unfavourable organisms can make their way into your small intestine. Over time, you can have an overgrowth of bacteria in the small intestine, which fires up your immune system. The resulting inflammation can fan the flames of acne breakouts.

What to do:

There are lots of reasons for hypochlorhydria (the fancy word for low stomach acid). These include advancing age, stress, zinc deficiency or long-term use of medications.

You can take steps to reduce your stress and boost your zinc intake (which we'll talk about chapter 6 and chapter 7 respectively). But you can't change your age, and you certainly shouldn't stop taking medication without first consulting your doctor.

Happily, there are a few techniques to support a healthy level of stomach acid:

- Eat something **bitter or acidic** at the start of your meal, as these trigger stomach acid production. Good choices include rocket leaves, chicory, radicchio and/or lemon juice. A simple starter salad could do the trick.
- Drink 1 tbsp of **apple cider vinegar** in a small glass of water, 20 minutes before each meal. Like stomach acid, apple cider vinegar has a low pH. Good, old-fashioned digestive bitters are another option that has a similar effect.
- Eat in a **relaxed state** and chew thoroughly, which you'll be doing if you've followed the previous point about putting your cutlery down between each bite.
- Follow the Okinawan principle of *hara hachi bu*, which means 'eat until you're **8 parts out of 10 full**'. Your digestion is better when you don't overwhelm your stomach.
- **Avoid drinking water** and other liquids with your meal, as this can dilute your stomach acid. Save any heavy drinking for half an hour after you've eaten.

Most people will benefit from these steps, but it's especially worth trying them if you find you feel full or belch soon after eating. You don't have to do them all—simply start with whichever suits you most.

The small intestine

What happens:
After two to four hours of churning, food passes through the lower valve of your stomach and enters your small intestine. Here, enzymes further break down food into its smallest-possible components, which are then absorbed through your intestinal wall.

What can go wrong:
The whole point of eating is to provide your body with the energy and nutrients it needs to carry out its daily functions.

That's why the small intestine is so important—it's where most of those nutrients get out of the digestive system and into the rest of the body. They then travel into the bloodstream to get to the body cells that need them most.

Three common states can compromise the function of the small intestine and contribute to acne:

1) Bacterial overgrowth

Small Intestine Bacterial Overgrowth (or SIBO for short) is a condition in which you have more bacteria in your small intestine than you should. As you learnt above, low stomach acid can contribute to this, but so can food poisoning, stress and antibiotic use.

People with acne rosacea (another type of acne characterised by flushing) are 13 times more likely to have SIBO than people without acne. SIBO is also believed to be behind up to 78% of IBS cases.

SIBO contributes to acne in two ways:

a) The bacteria eat your skin-supporting nutrients, including iron and vitamin B12.
b) The bacteria act as an irritant, causing the immune system to react. As 70% of your immune system is clustered around your gut, the resulting inflammation can spill over to parts of your body— including your face, chest and back.

What to do:

Symptoms such as diarrhoea, constipation, nausea, bloating and greasy stools may warrant SIBO investigation.

SIBO can be tricky to address, so it's best done with the support of a registered nutritional therapist. They may suggest you take a hydrogen breath test, which will show if there are misplaced bacteria lurking in your small intestine.

These bacteria feed on certain forms of carbohydrate, so it's a good idea to eat a low-fermentable-carbohydrate diet for eight to 12 weeks to 'starve' the bacteria. A nutritional therapist may also suggest you take probiotics and anti-microbials (you'll learn more about these in chapter 7).

2) Increased intestinal permeability

Nutrients get into your bloodstream by travelling through and between the cells in your small intestine wall. The 'gaps' between cells open up to let nutrients through, and then close up again. This is normal and healthy.

But problems arise when the gaps stay open for too long. This state of increased intestinal permeability (better known as 'leaky gut') means bigger food particles, bacteria and other unsavoury substances can get into your bloodstream. As with SIBO, your immune system doesn't like this—so it mounts an inflammatory response.

In one study, researchers took blood samples from patients with acne and patients with clear skin. They found that 65% of the blood from acne patients contained small bits of bacteria, indicating that they had leaky gut.

What to do:

If you follow all the principles outlined in this book, you'll naturally be eating and living in a way that promotes a strong gut barrier.

Here are the gut-healthy habits that we've covered so far:

- Balancing your blood sugar
- Eating high-quality protein
- Increasing your intake of omega-3 fats
- Minimising processed foods
- Reducing your toxic load
- Cutting down on alcohol and caffeine

And here are some that you'll learn in upcoming sections:

- Eating prebiotic fibre
- Enjoying a wide variety of colourful plant foods
- Making the most of probiotic foods
- Supplementing with key nutrients
- Experimenting with fasting
- Prioritising relaxation
- Improving your self-talk

Together, these have the power to dramatically reduce intestinal permeability. And minimising reactive foods—the next step—is the final piece of the puzzle.

3) Food sensitivities

Some people do react to specific foods. The most common culprits are dairy and wheat, but eggs, yeast, soy and corn can also cause problems. Gluten—found in wheat, but also rye and barley—can be troublesome too.

And yet there's a reason I've put this point last. You're much more likely to react to foods if you have compromised gut health, as described in the points above. This is because too-large bits of food end up in your bloodstream, where your immune system sees them as a foreign invader.

Yes, that's the immune system getting involved with your gut again. Are you noticing a theme here?

While some people are best off avoiding certain foods over the long-term, it's my experience that most people can eat small amounts of previously reactive foods once they've improved their gut health.

What to do:

If you suspect you have a food sensitivity, the best thing to do is to cut that food type out entirely (in the same way you may choose to eliminate dairy). It would be best if you could cut it out for three months, but three weeks can be enough to give an indication. While you cut out the food, introduce as many gut-supporting habits as you can.

To reintroduce, think '3 x 3'. After **three** months (or at least three weeks), eat the eliminated food **three** times in one day, and then wait **three** days. Here's how that might look in practice:

		Example 1	*Example 2*
Day 1	**Food**	*1 large egg x 3*	*1 slice wholemeal bread x 3*
	Symptoms?	*None*	*Bloating*
Day 2	*Symptoms?*	*None*	*Constipation*
Day 3	*Symptoms?*	*None*	*New pimple*
Tolerated?		✔	✗

It's best to test with a simple, unadorned form of the food. If you want to test wheat, for example, opt for toast rather than a fully loaded pizza base! If your skin doesn't react, you can eat that food once more. If your skin does react, eliminate it for another three months and try again.

You may feel you need to eliminate more than one food. In an ideal world, you'd reintroduce them all separately, leaving a couple of wash-out days before trying the next one. But sometimes that just isn't possible. If you notice symptoms, use it as an opportunity to be your own health detective. Eliminate and reintroduce until you've found that problematic food, and work out how much of it you can tolerate.

As ever, the most important thing is that you're eating a diet that's as diverse as possible. Your ideal diet will be as unique as you are.

The large intestine

What happens:

By the time your food gets to your large intestine, most of the nutrients have been absorbed. What's left is a large food residue mixture, known as a 'chyme'. Your body doesn't like to waste anything, so the large intestine takes water from the chyme and returns it to your cells. You excrete the remaining food waste products as faeces (poo).

What can go wrong:

Your large intestine isn't just a waste bin. It's home to a vibrant community known as your 'gut microbiome'.

That's right: you play host to bacteria, yeasts, viruses, protozoa and archaea. Together, these weigh 2kg, which is roughly the same as your brain.

It can be horrifying to learn you have these little critters inside you. But it's a very good thing! We don't yet know all the functions of the gut microbiome, but we do know it plays a role in:

- **Digesting your food**. Bacteria ferment the indigestible fibre in your food, releasing substances that help to heal your gut lining.
- **Regulating your immune system**. Bacteria are constantly talking to the immune cells clustered around your gut. That means they can influence inflammation.
- **Synthesising vitamins**. These bacteria also help to produce vitamin K and some B vitamins, which are essential for a healthy complexion.

What's interesting about this area of research is that it has thrown the notion of 'good bacteria' and 'bad bacteria' into question. We're coming to learn that it's more important to have a balance of bacteria and other microbes, as they all help to keep each other in check.

The problem is that many people's gut microbiomes are a little out of a shape. Poor diets, stress, medications, infection and toxins can diminish the number and types of bacteria in your gut microbiome—and this can wind up aggravating your skin. More than half of people with acne have been found to have a disrupted gut microbiome.

What to do:
Cultivating a balanced microbiome can help to calm your skin.

I'll be upfront: this takes patience and dedication. But it's worth it. I've observed that people who put effort into this find that their skin becomes less and less reactive over time.

There are four steps to making your microbiome as rich, diverse and resilient as possible:

1)   Eat prebiotic foods
A 'prebiotic' is a special type of fibre. You can't digest it—but your gut bacteria can. Eating prebiotic fibre provides the fuel for bacteria to flourish, enhancing the richness of your microbiome.

Boost your bacteria with the following:

Prebiotic food	Serving
Asparagus	4 spears
Chickpeas	½ cup, cooked
Garlic	1 clove
Green bananas	1 banana
Leeks	½ leek
Lentils	½ cup, cooked
Oats	1/3 cup
Onions	1 small onion

Aim to eat at least one of these foods daily. Be aware that suddenly eating large portions can cause flatulence, so it's best to work your way up to a full portion.

Beyond these specific foods, eating a wide variety of colourful fruits and vegetables will further enhance your microbiome. This is because each colour feeds a different sort of bacteria. Fill half your plate with vegetables at each meal, and challenge yourself to see how many colours you can fit in.

Further skin benefits of fibre
Aside from feeding your gut bacteria, fibre is important because it helps to keep you regular. This is an essential part of hormonal balance because used hormones are excreted when you go to the loo. And, as you learnt in chapter 2, happy hormones are essential for happy skin.

You should pass a well-formed stool at least once daily. I'll say this again because it is such a significant point—you should do a poo at least once a day!

If you go less than this or you have to strain, first increase your fibre and water intake and see if it makes a difference. If there's no change (or if it gets worse), see a registered nutritional therapist to investigate SIBO and other contributing factors.

2)   Eat probiotic foods

While prebiotics are fuel for friendly bacteria, probiotics are the friendly bacteria themselves.

We used to think that probiotics repopulated the gut microbiome. They can do this, but they also work in much more nuanced ways. Their other tactics include training the immune system, strengthening the intestinal barrier and stopping one bacterium from taking precedence (remember, diversity is key!).

It's this multi-faceted functioning that makes probiotics so good for your skin. Countless studies back this up, including one which showed that drinking fermented milk (kefir) reduced oiliness and improved acne in just 12 weeks.

Probiotic foods are most effective when you consume them regularly. Enjoy at least one of the below daily:

Probiotic food	Serving
Kefir	150ml
Kombucha	150ml
Natural live yoghurt	3 tbsp
Sauerkraut	2 tbsp
Kimchi	2 tbsp
Beet kvass	150ml

You'll notice that some of these foods are dairy-based. It's best to choose something else during your three-month dairy elimination, but after that, fermented dairy seems to be the most well-tolerated form. This may be because the process of fermentation naturally reduces levels of IGF-1—and less IGF-1 = less sebum.

3)   Experiment with fasting

Imagine your gut bacteria as a lawn. If you keep walking over the lawn, it will eventually wear down and become muddy. If you stop walking over the lawn, the grass has the chance to re-grow.

This is what happens to your gut bacteria when you eat. Food passing through can cause some types of bacteria to prosper at the detriment of others. Animal studies suggest that fasting helps all bacteria to prosper, increasing your diversity.

Just to recap: a diverse microbiome is a more balanced microbiome. A more balanced microbiome means more balanced skin.

Some people will tell you to go a full day without eating, but I find a more gentle, sustainable approach to fasting involves restricting your 'eating window' to 12 hours each day. In practice, this would mean eating your first bite of breakfast at 8am and your last bite of dinner by 8pm.

To bump up the effect, you can also minimise eating periods. Rather than grazing all day, enjoy three full meals and leave four to five hours between them. If you're eating to balance your blood sugar (as outlined in chapter 2), you should find that your appetite remains stable. You may even feel more energised.

As a side note, fasting also decreases those growth signals that are so problematic for acne-prone people, so it's a useful part of your toolbox. But please be sensible. If you have a history of disordered eating or suffer from diabetes, it's more important that you eat in a manner that keeps you physiologically and mentally balanced.

4) Relax

The fourth way to enhance your microbiome is to rest and unwind. Remember Stokes and Pillsbury's hypothesis that stress disrupts the gut microbiome? Yet again, they were right.

The 'gut-brain axis' is another new area of research. We can't yet explain all the mechanisms, but researchers have observed that stress reduces the diversity of gut bacteria.

Stress comes in many forms: mental, emotional, physical and even spiritual. We'll discuss stress more in chapter 6 but, for now, know that you need to make relaxation a priority.

Switching off isn't a luxury—it's a necessity. Your gut and your skin depend on it.

You've done it!

Phew! That was a long one, so well done for making it to the end.

You've worked your way through your entire digestion and learnt about possible acne triggers. If any of the points rang true for you, follow the advice in that section specifically, while incorporating as much as you can from the other sections too.

Next up: we're heading outside your body to explore your skin's barrier.

TAKE ACTION

Here's a recap of what to do:

✓ Only eat when sitting down, and put your cutlery down between each bite.

✓ Enjoy something bitter or acidic at the start of your meal, or try a tablespoon of apple cider vinegar in water 20 minutes before you eat. Stop eating when you're 80% full and save any heavy water-guzzling until afterwards.

✓ If you experience diarrhoea, bloating, constipation, nausea and/or fatty stools, see a registered nutritional therapist to investigate SIBO.

✓ If you think you have food sensitivities, eliminate the suspected food for at least three weeks. After elimination, test it by eating three portions of that food in one day, and then wait for three days to see if any symptoms appear. Use '3 x 3' to help you remember this process. You'll soon know if the food is contributing to your acne.

✓ Eat prebiotic and probiotic foods daily. And get into the habit of filling half your plate with colourful vegetables at every meal.

✓ Leave 12 hours between your last bite of dinner and your first bite of breakfast.

✓ Prioritise relaxation, both at mealtimes and during your day.

5. PROTECT YOUR SKIN'S BARRIER

Pay close attention if:
- *Your skin feels tight after cleansing*
- *You have a multi-step skincare routine*
- *Your skin is sensitive as well as acne-prone*
- *You regularly exfoliate your skin*
- *You go to bed with your make-up on*
- *You've tried oil cleansing*

QUICK READ
- What you put on your face is part of the acne puzzle, but it's important to address what you put inside your body first.
- Any products you use should complement your skin's pH and microbiome.
- You should avoid using products and substances that exacerbate the skin's inflammatory processes.

If you're anything like the other 85% of people who suffer from acne at some point in their life, you've no doubt spent a small fortune on cosmetics.

It can be tempting to think the next serum, the next spot cream or even the next four-step oil-cleansing method will be the answer to your prayers. But if you've picked up this book, chances are that none of those products or protocols lived up to their promises.

In my experience, it's only when you've addressed the inside (what you put *in* your body) that it's worth turning your attention to the outside (what you put *on* your skin). To understand why, picture a glass vase. No amount of polishing on the outside will make the vase sparkle and the flowers bloom. You have to make sure you put fresh water on the inside too.

As you've learnt, acne is a whole-body functioning issue. You've already tackled your hormones, your liver and your digestion, so you've taken huge strides to achieve clear skin.

And what you put on your skin is another important piece of the puzzle. You don't need to overhaul your entire skincare routine, but it will serve you to keep three questions in mind when choosing products. These are:

1)   Will this change my skin's pH?
2)   How will this affect my skin's microbiome?
3)   Can this influence my skin's inflammatory processes?

By this point, you know I like detail! Let's go through each in turn, and see why they're important considerations for conquering acne.

1)   <u>Will this change my skin's pH?</u>

Do you remember the concept of pH from your chemistry lessons at school? If not, here's a quick recap: pH stands for 'potential of hydrogen' or 'power of hydrogen' (believe it or not, the scientists can't agree). It's a scale that measures how acidic or how alkaline something is.

On this scale, 7 is neutral, anything below 7 is acidic and anything above 7 is alkaline. You may not think about it, but you come into contact with different pH values every day, such as:

pH	Example
0	Battery acid
1	Gastric acid
2	Lemon juice
3	Orange juice
4	Tomato juice
5	Black coffee

6	Milk
7	Pure water
8	Seawater
9	Baking soda
10	Milk of magnesia
11	Ammonia solution
12	Soapy water
13	Bleach
14	Liquid drain cleaner

You have a pH too—or, to be more specific, different areas of your body have different pH values. As you can see on the table, your gastric acid is highly acidic with a pH of 1. Your blood is ever-so-slightly alkaline with a pH of 7.35–7.45.

You may be surprised to learn that your skin is acidic. There is some variation between the genders but, on average, skin pH rests around 4.7. This 'acid mantle' plays a key role in the skin's barrier function, as well as providing the perfect conditions for the right bacteria to proliferate (more on this in the next section).

The problem is this acid mantle is easily disrupted. Again, as you can see on the table, soapy water has a pH of 12. If you wash your face with soapy water, you raise the pH of your facial skin for a few hours afterwards. If you keep washing your face with soapy water, you'll eventually induce a long-term change in your skin's pH.

But you'd never wash your face with ordinary soap! You know that. But you may not realise that many common skincare products also have a high (alkaline) pH. What that means is that with every cleanse, you're disrupting your acid mantle. This encourages bacterial overgrowth and inflammation, both of which exacerbate your acne.

It makes sense that people with acne have been found to have higher-than-optimal skin pH.

What to do:

The good news is that using the right products can help to repair the acid mantle. The secret is to become a smart consumer.

Use products with a pH of 4–5.5. Like your skin, these are slightly acidic, so they support a strong acid mantle. Sadly, we're not yet at the point where products list their pH on their label, but there are three ways you can find out:

1) **Look for the phrase 'pH balanced'.** This means the product's pH is close to that of natural skin.
2) **Buy some litmus strips and test it yourself.** Simply dip the strip into a sample of the product and see what colour it turns. This method isn't 100% accurate (and it will only work if there's water or 'aqua' in the product) but it's enough to give you an indication.
3) **Ask the manufacturer.** Companies know the pH of their products because they have to test it. If in doubt, get in touch with the customer care line (or sales representative) and ask.

Beyond this, choose products with minimal ingredients. Avoid cleansers with lots of fragrance and sodium lauryl sulphate (SLS), as these are known acid mantle-strippers. You can help your skin self-regulate if you use as few products as you feel comfortable with—so use it as an excuse to declutter your bathroom shelf.

2) <u>How will this affect my skin's microbiome?</u>

Your skin is home to bacteria, viruses, fungi and even mites. These begin to colonise your skin soon after you're born and by the time you reach adulthood, there are 1 million bacteria on every square centimetre of skin.

A commonly cited belief is that the bacterium Cutibacterium acnes (formerly known as Propionibacterium acnes) is one cause of acne. But newer findings suggest it's not that simple. Cutibacterium acnes is also dominant in people who don't have acne, and studies trying to find patterns between acne and the skin microbiome have been inconclusive.

This is probably because, like in the gut, it's not so much the specific bacteria that are important, but their balance.

Far from being unwelcome invaders, these microbes are essential because they help to educate the immune system in your skin. This means that cultivating a strong, well-balanced microbial ecosystem can help to create a calm, unreactive complexion.

What to do:

Let me be clear: there's still much we don't understand about these microbes. We don't even know what a 'normal' skin microbiome looks like. But we can follow some general principles to protect the skin's ecosystem:

Look after your acid mantle. Follow the steps in the previous section to maintain a slightly acidic pH, as this helps the right bacteria to flourish.

Be kind to your gut. Follow the steps in chapter 4 too! We don't know all the mechanisms, but we do know the gut microbiome and the skin microbiome talk. Some gut bacteria can even migrate to the skin.

Reduce oiliness. Certain bacteria feed on sebum. Don't worry: you don't need to continually blot your face. You'll naturally be reducing oiliness if you follow the advice in chapter 2.

Don't over-wash. A scientist in the 1930s discovered that when he washed his hands and arms, his skin microbial population decreased from 4.6 million to 1 million. Clean your face as little as you feel comfortable with, or ideally no more than twice a day. But…

Do go to bed with a bare face. Your microbiome recalibrates overnight, so you can give it a helping hand by making sure all make-up is out of the way.

Be gentle. Hot water and harsh rubbing with a towel can feel good, but your bacteria don't like it. Same goes for exfoliation—you don't need to do this more than once or twice a week.

Look out for preservatives. These are designed to kill bacteria. Be wary of products with a long shelf life.

Get dirty. Do some gardening, play with your pet or go on a long, muddy walk. Interaction with the natural world is a fun way to support microbial diversity.

Experiment with prebiotic/probiotic skincare. This is far from an exact science, but some people do find that it helps. Request some samples to see if it works for you.

With the correct pH and balanced microbes, you've already set the stage for happy skin. The final step is to modulate inflammation.

3) How will this affect my skin's inflammatory processes?

Together, the skin's pH and microbiome affect inflammatory processes. And one thing we do know is that inflammation is a key driver of acne.

This is an important point. Before, we thought that too much sebum, too many androgens, too many skin cells and the wrong skin bacteria led to spots, which then became inflamed. But now that's been turned on its head. Newer research shows that inflammation *causes* the excess cell growth that contributes to pimples.

What this means is that pre-existing inflammation may predispose you to developing acne.

The good news is that anything you do to dial down inflammation in your body—which is ultimately what the previous three chapters have been about—will have a knock-on effect on your skin. But you can also reduce inflammation by being selective about which products you put on your skin.

Two ingredients are especially worth mentioning:

ANTI-INFLAMMATORY: Tea tree oil
This essential oil from the Melaleuca alternifolia tree has been used as an antiseptic in Australia for centuries. One clinical trial found that it was just as effective as benzoyl peroxide at reducing acne lesions, and it had far fewer side effects.

It's best not to use tea tree oil neat on your skin. Instead, mix a single drop into your face cream at night and massage in (avoiding the eye area). It can take a few days to work, but it's a useful tactic to minimise a new breakout.

Try not to use tea tree oil every day. As well as being anti-inflammatory, it's also anti-microbial, which means overuse could affect your skin microbiome. You can use it every night for a few days and then take a break for a few days, or use it two to three times a week.

ANTI-INFLAMMATORY: Nicotinamide
Also known as niacinamide, this is a form of vitamin B3. One trial found that a nicotinamide gel was comparable to antibiotic gel at clearing acne. Interestingly, the oilier a person's skin, the better it worked.

This trial used a gel with 4% nicotinamide. You can easily buy serums and gels with that percentage and higher, so it's worth giving it a go. Most nicotinamide formulations are also moisturising, so you can use them every day.

One more ingredient is worth mentioning, but for the opposite reason:

PRO-INFLAMMATORY: Olive oil

Some people swear by oil cleansing—but I find it isn't the best approach for acne-prone skin. Not only are some oils comedogenic (meaning they block pores), they also contain substances that are pro-inflammatory when applied topically.

Case in point: oleic acid in olive oil. Your skin's immune system recognises this natural substance as a danger signal. Your immune cells start talking to each other to spread the message, starting a cascade of reactions that results in skin inflammation. Just to be clear, this only happens when you apply extra virgin olive oil to your face. It's still great acne-fighting food to eat.

The same principle applies to facial oils. Some contain 'danger signal' substances, and some contain fatty acids that feed the wrong type of microbes (including yeasts). The funny thing about this is that you can use a facial oil without problem in a cool climate, but as soon as you go to a hot and humid country, it contributes to breakouts. This is because the combination of humidity and excess fatty acids leads to microbial imbalance. And microbial imbalance sets the stage for—you guessed it—inflammation.

Experiment and see what works for you. If you use a facial oil and your skin hasn't reacted, great. If you're not sure, it can be worth replacing it with an oil-free moisturiser.

Chapter 6: done!

You are well on your way to achieving the skin you want. Not only have you learnt to optimise your hormones, digestion and liver function, you now know which types of cosmetics are best to help clear your complexion.

We're nearly there. Before we go on to the supplements that can give you extra support, let's talk about another crucial ingredient for happy skin: being kind to yourself.

TAKE ACTION

Here's a recap of what to do:

✓ Look for products that have a pH of 4–5.5. They'll often say 'pH balanced' but, if not, you can buy litmus strips and test them yourself. You can also ask the manufacturers.

✓ Try not to wash your face more than twice a day. To dry, pat it gently with a towel (rather than rubbing). Exfoliate no more than twice per week.

✓ Remove all make-up before you go to sleep.

✓ Look out for preservatives in your skincare—but don't be afraid to get dirty in the garden!

✓ Mix a drop of tea tree oil with your night-time moisturiser and rub it in, avoiding the eye area. Use a few times a week (but not every day).

✓ Try a product with nicotinamide. Look for at least a 4% solution.

✓ Avoid using olive oil on your face, and be cautious with facial oils. If you're certain a facial oil isn't contributing to your breakouts, great. If you're not sure, try an oil-free moisturiser instead.

6. TREAT YOURSELF WELL

Pay close attention if:
- *You're self-critical*
- *You lead a fast-paced life, or you don't get enough 'you' time*
- *You rarely get enough sleep*
- *You train hard at the gym*
- *You're addicted to your phone*

QUICK READ
- Food is powerful—but you can't ignore your lifestyle.
- The way you speak to yourself can have a physiological impact that drives acne.
- Relaxation, movement and sleep all play a role in cultivating clear skin.

Food is powerful. It can calm inflammation, balance hormones and support detoxification, all of which are essential for clear skin.

But food isn't the answer to everything. You are a complex and dynamic being, and your body constantly recalibrates to accommodate all aspects of your lifestyle. This includes your sleep patterns, your activity levels and your ability to relax.

If you're tempted to skip this section—thinking that you just want to know what to eat to beat your acne—I urge you to continue. For truly radiant skin, taking care of yourself is just as important as tweaking your diet.

Let's explore what this means in practice, and how you can streamline your non-dietary habits to further support your complexion.

Treat yourself well through…Relaxation and self-talk

Studies show that people with acne are more likely to feel depressed. Not only that, but they often have a reduced sense of self-worth. They even have less sex.

If you've been suffering from acne for a while, this will come as no surprise to you. Acne can shred your confidence and make you feel that you're not the person you want to be. That is not OK—and that's exactly why you've picked up this book.

But what might come as a surprise is that we don't know what drives this. The presumption has always been that self-consciousness about your skin makes you feel down—but could it that other physiological imbalances (including a disrupted gut microbiome) promote both acne and emotional distress?

We can't yet say for certain. It likely becomes a vicious circle: your skin gets you down, which disrupts your gut, which further inflames your skin, which makes you feel even more down. And if you're in this cycle, it's horrible.

Breaking this cycle is a vital part of clearing your skin. This is because, wherever it stems from, stress increases the hormone cortisol. Cortisol increases sebum, which (as you know by now) is one of the key ingredients for new pimples. It's no wonder a study found a correlation between daily stress and acne severity.

Calming your mind
Hang on, now you're stressed about not getting stressed! Please don't be. By working on your hormones, liver and gut, you're already balancing your body—so all that's left is to calm your mind. And a decreased stress response is a natural side effect of *minimising* effort and prioritising fun. There are two sides to this:

1) Being kind to yourself.
2) Finding your joy.

Let's explore both.

1) Be kind to yourself
I cannot emphasise this enough.

When you suffer from acne, it's easy to let it dominate your thoughts. You probably touch your face as soon as you wake up, tentatively feeling for what's sprouted overnight. Every time you look in a reflective surface, you scan your face for any bumps. You likely spend a good portion of your evening routine popping, squeezing and extracting.

You think about your acne so much that you now feel it defines you.

It doesn't define you—but it is down to you to take back control. And this starts with shifting your attention.

- Every time you look in the mirror, I want you to **focus on something you *do* like about your face**. Perhaps you've been complimented on your eyes or your smile. You may even just like your eyebrows. Whatever it is, look for that feature and make that the focus of your attention. This will take some practice, but its effect can be profound.

- Next the **picking, squeezing and extracting time has to go**. Let's be realistic: you know you're not supposed to squeeze spots, but neither are you willing to walk around with a whitehead on your face. I get it. But carefully extracting a spot with a sterilised needle, dabbing it with tea tree oil and moving on is one thing. Spending minutes (if not hours) scrutinising your face is another. I've found it to be true that what you focus on, grows. Save your mental real estate for something joyful (more on that in the next section).

- Finally, **tune into your self-talk**. It can be shocking to hear what you're saying to yourself. I'd wager you belittle your appearance, question your value and spitefully compare yourself to others. This has to stop. There are a few ways to tackle this, and different approaches chime with different people. Try some of these:
  a) Ask yourself whether you'd say that to a friend. If not, why are you saying it to yourself? Check yourself every time an insult rises up.
  b) Picture yourself as a child. What do you think that little person needs to hear? You're nourishing your body with good food, so nourish your mind with kind and loving thoughts.
  c) Imagine your mind as a gallery and your thoughts as paintings. If you didn't like a painting, you'd simply move on to the next one. You can do that with your thoughts too.
  d) Experiment with affirmations. 'I am enough' can be transformative. Affirmations aren't just about the words—the secret is to tune in to how the statement makes you feel when you're saying it.

e)   Escape the comparison trap. Social media is a showreel, and
you typically scroll through it during your most unexciting
moments. Find something else to do in your downtime.

You may be desperate to clear your skin, but you have to work on
clearing your mind too. Not only will this decrease your stress, but it will
also help you appreciate what's good about your skin (whether it's perfect
or not).

2) Find your joy

A huge part of relaxation is getting yourself out of your head and into your
body. This naturally draws your attention to the present moment, which is a
known tactic for reducing stress.

We've all experienced that state of 'flow'. It's where you're so focused
that time passes without you realising it. You feel more alive, and maybe
even elated.

This is more powerful when it's an active rather than a passive activity.
You may think that watching TV relaxes you, for example, but you may not
have unlocked how a calligraphy session can make you feel. For clues about
what can get you into flow, think back to what you used to like doing as a
child. Maybe dancing is your thing, or perhaps you once had a passion for
painting. The sweet spot for flow is where you feel simultaneously
challenged and skilled.

To boost your relaxation and enhance your sense of joy, I want you to
get into that state of flow every day. It needn't be for long: just 15 minutes
is enough to have an effect. Dedicate whatever time you can afford.

Remember: reduced stress means reduced cortisol. Reduced cortisol
means calmer skin.

The options are endless but, if you need inspiration, here are a few
suggestions to get you started:

- Play with your pet
- Read your favourite book
- Pick up that instrument you once played
- Have a go at meditation
- Try journalling
- Put on your favourite song and dance
- Go for a country walk
- Book a class in something you'd like to try
- Spend time with people you love (this one is hugely important)
- Cook a new recipe

A side effect of focusing on joy is distracting yourself from what bothers you. And how freeing would it be to not constantly worry about your skin?

Treat yourself well through...Moving your body

Exercise and acne is a delicate balance: you want neither too much nor too little, but just the right amount.

Too little exercise contributes to insulin resistance, which leads to higher levels of insulin in your blood. As you learnt in chapter 2, too much insulin drives the production of acne-promoting androgens. But too much exercise isn't good either. The physiological stress of overtraining can raise cortisol, which increases sebum, and it can also exacerbate leaky gut.

A healthy, sustainable level of exercise does support clear skin. This is because it:

- Enhances insulin sensitivity
- Reduces inflammation
- Helps you destress

Just the right amount

But how do you know what's the right amount for you? The first step is to be honest with yourself. If you have a niggling feeling that you could up your physical activity, it's probably true. On the flip side, if you're beginning to wonder if your intense gym routine is contributing to your fatigue and aching joints, you may wish to think about scaling back.

I am no exercise expert, but I have found two principles to be helpful:

1) Exercise should leave you feeling more, not less, energised.
There's nothing like the endorphin rush after a good run or the joy of a fast-paced game of tennis with friends. You may feel weary afterwards, but it's a good kind of weary—and it makes you feel like you want to make the most of your day.

Pushing yourself through your fourth cross-fit session of the week— while wondering how on earth you're going to muster the energy to get through a full working day—is quite different. Give yourself the grace to listen to your body. Chances are, it's telling you something.

2) Exercise should fit into the context of your lifestyle.
I've said it before but it's worth repeating: you are a dynamic being. You can't be expected to maintain the same pace of activity every day because so many factors contribute to your energy levels.

If you're having an especially stressful week at work, an intense HIIT session might not be the best option for you. You may find more stress relief in a relaxing yoga routine. If you're on holiday and you've spent days lounging by the pool, a sweaty round of circuits may be just what you need to feel invigorated.

Guidelines dictate that to stay healthy, adults should do at least 150 minutes of moderate-intensity exercise each week such as cycling or brisk walking, along with two sessions of strength exercises. If the exercise is more vigorous, you can do as little as 75 minutes weekly. Bear this in mind and try different forms of exercise, choosing the type of movement that suits on a particular day. Like your food, go for variety.

Treat yourself well through...Sleep

You know that you should take your make-up off before you go bed, but have you ever considered how the act of sleeping itself can help your complexion?

Sleep is deeply restorative for your mind and your body, and yet most of us aren't getting enough. A survey conducted in 2016 found that the typical Briton undersleeps by an hour every night. Over a week, that constitutes a sleep debt of 7 hours—almost a whole night's sleep.

If we look at mechanisms in the body, sleep debt can aggravate acne in a few ways:

- **It raises cortisol.** Yes, that's cortisol creeping up again. As you now know, cortisol fans acne flames because it increases sebum production.
- **It increases appetite.** A lack of sleep makes you more likely to reach for that sugary energy hit. Sleep deprivation also increases the amount of insulin you release after eating, further contributing to excess androgens and sebum.
- **It can make you moody and emotional**. Remember Stokes and Pillsbury from chapter 4? If they're to be believed, emotional states can alter the gut microbiome—exacerbating the inflammation that also drives acne.

How to maximise your sleep
Sleep is an important part of your toolbox for clear skin. But let's be realistic: sometimes those ideal eight hours just aren't possible. Perhaps you're caring for small children, or perhaps you have late nights because you're having fun.

Though you can't expect yourself to have perfect slumber every night, you can take steps to maximise high-quality hours of kip so that your overall sleep debt diminishes. This involves practising a set of sleep-promoting behaviours and habits known as 'sleep hygiene'.

Here's what to do:

Stick to a routine. Your body prefers you to go to bed and wake up at roughly the same time each day. Adhere to this as much as possible—but don't feel you need to miss out on social occasions. After all, happiness is good for your skin too!

Create a wind-down ritual. Find out what relaxes you and commit to doing it for half an hour before bed. This could be journalling, having a bath or enjoying a good, old-fashioned book.

Drink valerian tea an hour before bedtime. A cousin of chamomile, this has a long tradition of use as a sleep aid. Please note, you shouldn't drive after drinking this.

Cultivate your sleep environment. Keep your bedroom cool and dark, and open the window if possible. Invest in a comfortable mattress and pillows (it's worth it, as you spend a third of your life in bed).

Limit your screen time. Screens emit blue light that interferes with the production of melatonin, your sleep hormone. In an ideal world, you'd turn off all screens two hours before going to bed. If that isn't possible (and for most people, it isn't), switch your device to its 'night' setting so that it emits less blue light.

Make the bedroom a phone-free zone. This can be transformative. If you can't avoid screens for an hour or two before bed, at least keep them out of the bedroom—you'll be amazed at how much earlier you turn the light off. Buy an alarm clock if necessary.

See the sun. Exposure to natural light helps to create a robust circadian rhythm, so see the sun as soon as you can after you wake up. If you can head outside for half an hour, even better.

Avoid exercising too close to bedtime. This can be stimulating, making it hard for you to drop off. Try to leave four hours between exercising and going to bed.

There are also a few dietary habits that can help with sleep, which you'll recognise from previous chapters:

Eat intelligently. A well-balanced meal will keep your blood sugar steady overnight. Flip back to chapter 2 to re-read the principles of blood-sugar balancing.

Be mindful about caffeine intake. We all metabolise caffeine differently, but most people benefit from limiting coffee and tea in the afternoon. Head to chapter 3 for the tell-tale signs that you're drinking too much caffeine.

Drink sensibly. You also learnt in chapter 3 that it's best to save alcohol for special occasions. If you do drink, try to have your last sip by 10pm. You'll make life easier for your liver and you'll sleep better too.

You don't have to do all of this every day—simply embrace as many of these habits as you can. High-quality sleep will not only make you feel better, but it's another thread in the fabric of great skin.

Nearly there!
Self-kindness is essential for everyone, but especially for people struggling with skin issues. You've taken great strides by choosing nourishing foods and gentle cosmetics, and now you've learnt how to turn your mind, movement and sleep to your advantage too.

These lay the foundations for good health and glowing skin. Only when these are in place can we add the cherry on top: supplemental nutrients.

Read on to discover which supplements could be the final piece in your acne puzzle.

TAKE ACTION
Here's a recap of what to do:

- ✓ Every time you look in the mirror, focus on something you like about your face.

- ✓ Phase out the minutes (or hours) you spend picking, squeezing and extracting—save your time for something more joyful.

- ✓ Tune into your self-talk. If you wouldn't say something to a friend, why are you saying it to yourself?

✓ Think back to what you used to like doing as a child, and get into a state of 'flow' for 15 minutes each day. Relaxation is a necessity, not a luxury.

✓ Find forms of movement you enjoy and do them for a total of 75–150 minutes each week. Make sure they leave you feeling more (not less) energised.

✓ Prioritise your sleep through practising sleep hygiene. This includes creating a wind-down routine, avoiding screens for two hours before bed and making your bedroom as comfortable as possible.

7. SUPPLEMENT WISELY

Pay close attention if:
- *You've worked hard to optimise your diet*
- *You prioritise movement, sleep and relaxation*
- *You suspect your gut needs some extra support*
- *Your acne is noticeably worse before your period*
- *You have known nutritional deficiencies*

QUICK READ
- Supplements should only ever complement sound dietary and lifestyle habits.
- Supplements can be potent, but they don't work overnight. Expect to take them for a minimum of three months.
- Choose the highest-quality supplements you can afford.

At the beginning of this book, we spoke about the trap of monotherapy—that is, believing one intervention will change a multi-factorial condition. As you've learnt, your body doesn't work like that. And yet how many times have you wished that taking a pill could make your acne disappear?

Many people approach supplements in this manner. They hear a certain nutrient or herb can help, so they start taking it—and then become frustrated when they don't see results in a few days. But supplements aren't like drugs: they work more subtly and more slowly.

To make the most of supplements, you need to:

1) **Choose high-quality formulations**. There's a world of difference between a cheap, high-street supplement and a professional-grade formulation. Like food, it serves you to pay for quality because your body will get more from it. For a list of my favourite supplement brands, turn to Appendix II.
2) **Be patient.** Supplements don't work overnight. You should expect to take them for three to four months before assessing their effectiveness.
3) **Use them appropriately.** The clue is in the name: supplements should only ever complement good foundational habits.

That last point is especially important. To understand this, picture a house. Your lifestyle habits (sleep, relaxation and movement) are the foundations. Your healthy diet is the bricks and mortar. Only when these are in place can you begin to think about the furnishings—supplements. After all, buying curtains before you've built your walls would be a waste of time and money.

Making supplements work for you

It's still preferable to get your nutrients from food, which is why I've listed the food sources of the below nutrients where appropriate. Eat these foods as well as taking the supplement.

You don't need to take all of these. The first four are appropriate for most people, but use what you've learnt in the preceding chapters to work out which of the rest could be helpful for you.

Neither do you need to take them forever. Commit to taking them for three to four months to begin with, and then gradually decrease the dose. If your skin is fine, stop taking the supplements but continue to eat the nutrient-rich foods. If you notice your skin reacts, take the full dose for another three months and then try again. Most people find they can come off supplements within a year.

Some of these supplements have been found to reduce acne in clinical trials, while others are worth trying because of how they influence certain pathways in the body. As ever, be guided by the evidence, but don't be afraid to experiment and see what works for you.

Please note, some supplements can interact with medications. If you're taking prescription medication or oral contraceptives, or if you're pregnant or breastfeeding, please check with your doctor before taking any supplements.

Top choices for acne

Most people benefit from all four of these, but feel free to start with a couple.

Zinc
Where to find it in food: meat, shellfish, chickpeas, lentils, nuts, seeds

Why it helps: studies show that acne sufferers tend to have lower levels of zinc in their blood and skin. A few clinical trials have found that supplementing with zinc reduces acne, likely because it reduces sebum and has an anti-inflammatory effect.

Supplement dose: **15mg zinc, twice a day with food** (do not take on an empty stomach, as this can cause nausea). The forms zinc picolinate, zinc gluconate or zinc sulphate are best, so read labels closely. If you take zinc for more than three months, you must also supplement with 1–2mg copper daily to avoid imbalances.

Fish oil
Where to find it in food: salmon, mackerel, anchovies, sardines, herring

Why it helps: docosahexaenoic acid (DHA) and eicosapentaenoic acid (EPA), two omega-3 fats in fish oil, are known to have anti-inflammatory effects. One study showed that supplementing with 2g EPA and DHA reduced the number of pimples in acne sufferers after ten weeks.

Supplement dose: **5ml liquid or 2 capsules fish oil, once a day**. Look for a formulation that has roughly equal amounts of DHA and EPA.

Saccharomyces boulardii
Where to find it in food: no food sources

Why it helps: one study found that a particular strain of friendly yeast ('Saccharomyces cerevisiae var boulardii Hansen CBS 5926') improved acne in 80% of sufferers. Saccharomyces boulardii supplements have slightly different strains, but they all support microbial balance—which has a knock-on effect on acne.

Supplement dose: **5 billion colony forming units (CFUs), twice a day**. High-quality formulations will include the CFU value on the label. Do not take Saccharomyces boulardii if you have an allergy to yeast.

Vitamin D

Where to find it in food: oily fish, seafood and egg yolks. Your skin also makes vitamin D during sensible exposure to sunlight

Why it helps: one study found that vitamin D tends to be lower in acne sufferers. This important vitamin modulates your immune system, as well as supporting a strong gut barrier.

Supplement dose: **10–25mcg vitamin D3, once a day**. If you live in the northern hemisphere, it's good practice to take vitamin D during the winter months. But it is possible to take too much. You can check your blood levels by buying an at-home vitamin D test kit.

For further gut support

If you feel your gut needs a helping hand, choose a probiotic and either berberine or oil of oregano. Cod liver oil can replace fish oil supplements.

Probiotics

Where to find it in food: sauerkraut, kefir, kimchi, kombucha, natural live yoghurt

Why it helps: probiotics don't always repopulate your gut microbiome, but they do help to modulate it. A study conducted in the 1960s found that Lactobacillus bulgaricus and Lactobacillus acidophilus species can help acne, though we can't yet say which strains are best.

Supplement dose: **20–50 billion CFUs, once a day**. Look for a probiotic with a combination of strains.

Cod liver oil

Where to find it in food: cod liver!

Why it helps: as well as providing omega-3 fats, cod liver oil is a valuable source of pre-formed vitamin A (retinol). Vitamin A plays a key role in skin health—so it's not surprising that one study found that acne sufferers tend to have lower levels of it.

Supplement dose: **1 tsp, once a day**. Buy the highest-grade cod liver oil you can afford. If you're taking this, you don't need to take fish oil too. **Please note, pregnant women should not take cod liver oil.**

Berberine
Where to find it in food: barberries

Why it helps: one fascinating study found that taking barberry extract (a source of berberine) reduce inflamed spots in just four weeks. Berberine is a potent acne-fighter: it modulates bacteria, reduces testosterone and improves insulin sensitivity.

Supplement dose: **500mg, twice a day**. Don't take this for longer than three months at a time. Take a month's break, and then go back to it if necessary.

Oil of oregano
Where to find it in food: fresh oregano

Why it helps: like berberine, oil of oregano is naturally anti-microbial. It's one of the first supplements I turn to for supporting healthy, balanced gut bacteria.

Supplement dose: **300mg, twice a day**. Like berberine, don't take this for longer than three months at a time. Take a month's break, and then go back to it if necessary.

For further hormonal support

If your acne is worse before your period, vitamin B6 can be a helpful option. If you have other signs of high androgens (such as excess body hair, or a thinning of hair on the head), saw palmetto can be worth trying.

Vitamin B6 (Pyridoxine)
Where to find it in food: chicken, fish, eggs, wholegrains

Why it helps: Two trials—one conducted in the 1940s and another in the 1970s—found that supplementing with vitamin B6 reduced premenstrual acne and oiliness. Vitamin B6 is known to help other symptoms of PMS too, especially when combined with magnesium.

Supplement dose: **50mg, once a day**. It's best to find a formulation that contains other B vitamins too, or one that combines vitamin B6 with magnesium.

Saw palmetto
Where to find it in food: no food sources

Why it helps: this herb prevents testosterone from turning into the more potent DHT. This helps to reduce acne-driving sebum.

Supplement dose: **150mg, twice a day**. It's best to take this with food.

For further liver support

If you suspect your toxic load is playing a role in your acne, try the below.

Liver formula
Where to find this in food: refer back to chapter 3 to see liver-supporting foods.

Why it helps: in chapter 3, we also looked at a 1950s Japanese study that found liver-supporting nutrients could improve acne. There has been little research confirming this since, though I have found it to be helpful clinically.

Supplement dose: **1–2 capsules, daily**. Look for a formulation that contains ingredients such as n-acetylcysteine, milk thistle, alpha-lipoic acid and amino acids such as taurine, glycine and l-methionine.

You've done it!
You've finished! In your journey to improve your skin, you've addressed your hormones, liver, digestive system, movement, sleep and mind. You also know which supplements can provide extra support.

Not only will these habits positively influence your skin, but they'll also boost your health as a whole. You should congratulate yourself on your commitment to looking after yourself from the inside-out.

Feeling overwhelmed? Don't worry! In the final chapter, we'll recap everything you've learnt so you can implement it in your everyday life.

TAKE ACTION

Here's a recap of what to do:

✓ *If you're taking prescription medication or oral contraceptives, or if you're pregnant or breastfeeding, please check with your doctor before taking any supplements.*

✓ Choose 2 or more of the following:
  o **Zinc**: 15mg, twice a day. Take with food.
  o **Fish oil**: 5ml or 2 capsules, once a day. Look for a formulation with an equal amount of EPA and DHA.
  o **Saccharomyces boulardii**: 5 billion CFUs, twice a day. Do not take this if you have an allergy to yeast.
  o **Vitamin D**: 10–25mcg vitamin D3, once a day. Test your levels before taking this.

✓ If you feel your gut needs extra support, take 1 or 2 of the following:
  o **Probiotics**: 20–50 billion CFUs, once a day. Look for a multi-strain formulation.
  o **Cod liver oil**: 1tsp, once a day. You don't need to take this if you're already taking fish oil.
  o **Berberine**: 500mg, twice a day. Don't take this for more than 3 months at a time.
  o **Oil of oregano**: 300mg, twice a day. You don't need to take this if you're already taking berberine.

✓ Try these for extra hormonal support:
  o **Vitamin B6**: 50mg, once a day. This is worth trying if your acne is worse before your period.
  o **Saw palmetto**: 150mg, twice a day. This can help if you have other signs of high androgens (such as excess body hair).

✓ If you feel your liver needs a helping hand, take 1–2 capsules of a **liver-supporting supplement** daily. Look for a formulation that contains n-acetylcysteine, milk thistle, alpha lipoic acid and amino acids.

✓ Take the supplements for 3–4 months. After that, gradually reduce the dose and see how your skin fares. If it worsens, take a full dose for another 3 months and try again. If your skin is fine, you can phase out the supplements.

✓ As well as taking supplements, eat foods that are rich in the nutrients you're looking to replace.

8. MAKE HAPPY SKIN A HABIT

Congratulations! Change isn't easy, but you've taken the first step by reading this book.

I hope that you now see that, despite the current limitations of acne research, there's so much you can do to support your skin. Be guided by what we do know, but don't be afraid to take steps to see what works for you.

I also hope this book has released you from the maddening belief that one pill, one food or one supplement is going to stamp out your acne—if only you could find it. The truth is acne is a multi-factorial condition and it needs a multi-pronged approach.

The good news? You're well on your way to making that happen.

How long is it going to take?

This is the first question anyone asks. The honest answer is that there's no set time period, as we're all biochemically unique and our bodies respond differently.

What I can tell you is that your gut lining regenerates roughly every five days. Your skin renews itself every 28 days. What that means is that if you're committed to trying what you've learnt, you can expect to notice a difference within a few weeks. Most people see significant change after three months.

Now let me be straight with you: people see dramatic results by following this approach, but I wouldn't want to guarantee that you'll never see another pimple again. Your body is a brilliant entity, but it's not immune to the challenges of life.

What I can promise is that by following these steps, you'll feel more in control of your skin health. You'll learn what triggers your acne and you'll know how to manage it. With a little effort and patience, breakouts will no longer dominate your life—and if pimples do occur, they'll be rare and insignificant.

What I can also promise is that if you take these steps in your stride, you'll support your physical health and mental wellbeing. When you have those, clear skin is the cherry on top.

<u>Change your skin and change your life</u>

You've learnt a great deal in the previous chapters, but the most important part is that you put it into action.

You don't have to do all of this forever. Depending on your acne severity, it will serve you to follow the guidelines closely for the first three months. After that, flex it and see what works for you. See these changes as a way of conversing with your complexion—if it likes an action you're taking, it will show you.

I've included a summary of the guidelines below. What can you do today? Start there, and work your way up to including further habits. For more detail, flip back to the relevant chapter.

My goal is that you come to see what I hinted at in the first chapter: acne can be an opportunity. Don't get me wrong—I know acne can be deeply distressing and I'm not trying to dismiss that. But if having acne pushes you to nourish your body, change your self-talk and ultimately be kind to yourself, it can wind up having a positive effect on the rest of your life.

Here's to feeling great, inside and out.

Principle	Guidelines	Actions
Help your hormones	Balance your blood sugar	• Eliminate sugary foods and drinks • Choose high-fibre carbohydrates • Eat a source of protein and/or healthy fat with every meal and snack
	Be mindful about dairy	• Eliminate all dairy for three months • Reintroduce dairy, one type at a time, and monitor for reactions • Try goat's and/or sheep's dairy to see if you tolerate it better
	Eat the right fats	• Use small amounts of butter and/or coconut oil in cooking • Enjoy olive oil, avocado, nuts or seeds with each meal • Eat oily fish two to three times per week • Avoid all forms of trans fat
Look after your liver	Maximise your detoxification	• Eat liver-supporting foods such as lean protein, cruciferous vegetables, berries, flaxseed, grapefruit, beetroot, garlic and green tea
	Minimise your toxic load	• Stop smoking, cut down on your use of plastic, and replace your cleaning products and cosmetics with organic versions • If you drink alcohol, save it for special occasions • Choose organic food as

		much as you can
Be kind to your gut	Chew your food well	• Only eat when sitting down, and put your cutlery down after each bite
	Optimise your stomach acid	• Eat something bitter or acidic at the start of your meal, or try digestive bitters • Eat in a relaxed state • Eat until you're satisfied, but not stuffed • Avoid drinking water and other liquids with your meal (drink a glass 30 minutes before or afterwards)
	Support your gut integrity	• Investigate food intolerances by eliminating suspected food for three weeks to three months • Reintroduce that food and monitor for reactions—you'll soon know if it's causing you problems • If you suffer from constipation, diarrhoea, nausea, bloating and/or greasy stools, consider seeing a nutritionist to investigate SIBO
	Cultivate your friendly bacteria	• Eat prebiotic foods such as asparagus, lentils and oats • Eat probiotic food such as sauerkraut, kimchi, kefir and kombucha • Experiment with intermittent fasting, but only if it's feasible for you

		• Take a moment to relax every day
Protect your skin's barrier	Look after your skin's pH	• Choose skincare products that have a pH of 4–5.5 • Avoid products that contain SLS and/or lots of fragrance
	Consider your skin's microbiome	• Try not to wash your face more than twice a day • Remove your make-up before you go to bed • Exfoliate no more than twice a week, and don't rub your face too vigorously with your towel • Get dirty in the natural world: do some gardening, play with your pet or go for a country walk • Avoid skincare products with a long shelf life
	Minimise inflammatory processes	• Try adding one to two drops of tea tree oil to your night-time moisturiser • Experiment with using topical nicotinamide (a 4% solution or higher) • Avoid using olive oil on your face • If your acne is flaring, reconsider the use of other facial oils
Treat yourself well	Be kind to yourself	• Every time you look in the mirror, focus on something you like about your face • Phase out the time you spend picking, squeezing

		and eliminating • Tune in to your self-talk. Ask yourself, 'Would I say that to a friend?'
	Find your joy	• Think back to what you liked doing as a child—are you missing out on a hobby? • Get into a state of 'flow' for at least 15 minutes every day
	Move your body	• Find a form of movement you enjoy, and do it for 75–150 minutes every week • Adapt your exercise intensity to your life by switching between restorative and challenging movement
	Prioritise your sleep	• Try to go to bed and get up at the same time each day • Create a wind-down ritual • Make your bedroom as comfortable as possible • Keep your phone out of your bedroom • Expose yourself to natural light as soon as you can after you wake up
Supplement wisely	Take targeted nutrients	• Consider supplementing with two or more of the following: zinc, fish oil, saccharomyces boulardii, vitamin D • If you feel your gut needs further support, take probiotics. You can also take oil of oregano or berberine

		• You can also take cod liver oil instead of fish oil (as long as you're not pregnant) • If your skin is noticeably worse before your period, trying taking vitamin B6 or saw palmetto • For further liver support, take a liver formulation
	Use supplements appropriately	• If you're taking prescription medication or oral contraceptives, or if you're pregnant or nursing, please check with your doctor before taking any supplements • Optimise your diet and lifestyle before adding in supplements • Expect to take supplements for at least three months before assessing their effect • Choose the highest-quality formulations you can afford

Refer to the list as often as you need. As time goes on, you'll find these habits become a way of life.

Happy skin is within your grasp. As Hippocrates, the father of modern medicine, said more than 2,000 years ago:

"Healing is a matter of time, but it's sometimes also a matter of opportunity."

APPENDIX I

Food groups

Please note, the examples are not exhaustive—they're listed to give you inspiration.

Fat	Fat & Protein	Protein	Protein & Carbohydrate	Carbohydrate
Avocado **Butter** **Oils** e.g. extra virgin olive oil, coconut oil, avocado oil, hemp seed oil	**Dairy** e.g. full-fat milk, yoghurt, cheese (including sheep's and goat's) **Nuts** e.g. almonds, pecans, cashews, pistachios	**Eggs** **Fish** e.g. cod, haddock, hake **Meat** e.g. beef, lamb, venison, pork	**Pulses** e.g. lentils, chickpeas, kidney beans, butter beans, haricot beans **Quinoa**	**Fruit** e.g. apples, pears, blueberries, raspberries, plums, apricots, kiwis, oranges **Non-starchy vegetables** e.g. kale, broccoli, cabbage, cauliflower, spinach, onion, garlic, peppers, aubergine

Fat (cont.)	Fat & Protein (cont.)	Protein (cont.)	Protein & Carbohydrate (cont.)	Carbohydrate (cont.)
	Oily fish e.g. salmon, mackerel, sardines **Seeds** e.g. pumpkin, sunflower, sesame, flaxseed, chia seeds	**Poultry** e.g. chicken, turkey, duck, goose **Shellfish** e.g. crab, crayfish, prawns, squid **Tofu**		**Starchy vegetables** e.g. potatoes, sweet potatoes, squash, parsnips, carrots **Whole grains** e.g. brown rice, wild rice, oats, barley, rye, millet

APPENDIX II

<u>Preferred supplement brands</u>

I often turn to these brands because they offer sophisticated, evidence-based formulations. Some products are available on the high-street, while others you'll need to order through registered nutritional therapist.

Many of these brands have detailed documents on each of their formulations, so don't be shy about asking for more information.

Allergy Research Group

Bare Biology

Bio-Kult

BioMedica

Biotics Research Corporation

Designs for Health

Nordic Naturals

Nutri Advanced

Pure Encapsulations

Symprove

Terranova

Wild Nutrition

APPENDIX III

References

I read all of these papers during the creation of this book—and there are many, many more on the topic of food and acne. Head to ncbi.nlm.nih.gov/pubmed to find them.

Chapter 1 – Acne, Science and You

Burris J, Rietkerk W, Woolf K. Acne: the role of medical nutrition therapy. J Acad Nutr Diet. 2013;113(3):416-30.

Carlos-reyes Á, López-gonzález JS, Meneses-flores M, et al. Dietary Compounds as Epigenetic Modulating Agents in Cancer. Front Genet. 2019;10:79.

Fiedler F, Stangl GI, Fiedler E, Taube KM. Acne and Nutrition: A Systematic Review. Acta Derm Venereol. 2017;97(1):7-9.

Kaimal S, Thappa DM. Diet in dermatology: revisited. Indian J Dermatol Venereol Leprol. 2010;76(2):103-15.

Kucharska A, Szmurło A, Sińska B. Significance of diet in treated and untreated acne vulgaris. Postepy Dermatol Alergol. 2016;33(2):81-6.

Sackett D, Strauss S, Richardson W, et al. Evidence-Based Medicine: How to Practice and Teach EBM.2nd ed. Churchill Livingstone; Edinburgh: 2000

Skroza N, Tolino E, Semyonov L, et al. Mediterranean diet and familial dysmetabolism as factors influencing the development of acne. Scand J Public Health. 2012;40(5):466-74.

Tan AU, Schlosser BJ, Paller AS. A review of diagnosis and treatment of acne in adult female patients. Int J Womens Dermatol. 2018;4(2):56-71.

Tilles G. Acne pathogenesis: history of concepts. Dermatology (Basel). 2014;229(1):1-46.

Zouboulis CC, Katsambas A, Kligman AM. Pathogenesis and Treatment of Acne and Rosacea. Springer; 2014.

Chapter 2 – Help Your Hormones

Adebamowo CA, Spiegelman D, Berkey CSl. Milk consumption and acne in teenaged boys. J Am Acad Dermatol 2008; 58:787-93.

Benmoussa A, Provost P. Milk MicroRNAs in Health and Disease. Compre Rev Food Sci and Food Safe. 2019;18(3):1-20

Clatici VG, Voicu C, Voaides C, Roseanu A, Icriverzi M, Jurcoane S. Diseases of Civilization - Cancer, Diabetes, Obesity and Acne - the Implication of Milk, IGF-1 and mTORC1. Maedica (Buchar). 2018;13(4):273-281.

Danby FW. Nutrition and acne. Clin Dermatol. 2010;28(6):598-604.

James MJ, Gibson RA, Cleland LG. Dietary polyunsaturated fatty acids and inflammatory mediator production. Am J Clin Nutr. 2000;71(1 Suppl):343S-8S.

Juhl CR, Bergholdt HKM, Miller IM, Jemec GBE, Kanters JK, Ellervik C. Dairy Intake and Acne Vulgaris: A Systematic Review and Meta-Analysis of 78,529 Children, Adolescents, and Young Adults. Nutrients. 2018;10(8)

Katta R, Desai SP. Diet and dermatology: the role of dietary intervention in skin disease. J Clin Aesthet Dermatol. 2014;7(7):46-51.

Kumari R, Thappa DM. Role of insulin resistance and diet in acne. Indian J Dermatol Venereol Leprol. 2013;79(3):291-9.

Melnik BC. Evidence for acne-promoting effects of milk and other insulinotropic dairy products. Nestle Nutr Workshop Ser Pediatr Program. 2011;67:131-45.

Melnik BC. Dietary intervention in acne: Attenuation of increased mTORC1 signaling promoted by Western diet. Dermatoendocrinol. 2012;4(1):20-32.

Melnik BC. Diet in acne: further evidence for the role of nutrient signalling in acne pathogenesis. Acta Derm Venereol. 2012;92(3):228-31.

Melnik BC. Linking diet to acne metabolomics, inflammation, and comedogenesis: an update. Clin Cosmet Investig Dermatol. 2015;8:371-88.

Melnik BC. Milk--A Nutrient System of Mammalian Evolution Promoting mTORC1-Dependent Translation. Int J Mol Sci. 2015;16(8):17048-87.

Melnik BC. The TRAIL to acne pathogenesis: let's focus on death pathways. Exp Dermatol. 2017;26(3):270-272.

Melnik BC. Milk disrupts p53 and DNMT1, the guardians of the genome: implications for acne vulgaris and prostate cancer. Nutr Metab (Lond). 2017;14:55.

Melnik BC. Acne vulgaris: The metabolic syndrome of the pilosebaceous follicle. Clin Dermatol. 2018;36(1):29-40.

Melnik BC, Schmitz G. Exosomes of pasteurized milk: potential pathogens of Western diseases. J Transl Med. 2019;17(1):3.

Ottaviani M, Camera E, Picardo M. Lipid mediators in acne. Mediators Inflamm. 2010;2010

Pappas A. The relationship of diet and acne: A review. Dermatoendocrinol. 2009;1(5):262-7.

Romańska-Gocka K, Woźniak M, Kaczmarek-skamira E, Zegarska B. The possible role of diet in the pathogenesis of adult female acne. Postepy Dermatol Alergol. 2016;33(6):416-420.

Smith RN, Braue A, Varigos GA, Mann NJ. The effect of a low glycemic load diet on acne vulgaris and the fatty acid composition of skin surface triglycerides. J Dermatol Sci. 2008;50(1):41-52.

Tan JKL, Stein gold LF, Alexis AF, Harper JC. Current Concepts in Acne Pathogenesis: Pathways to Inflammation. Semin Cutan Med Surg. 2018;37(3S):S60-S62.

Chapter 3 – Look After Your Liver

Aikawa A, Mihara J, Tanida T, Tsukada S. The effects of glucuronic acid on acne vulgaris. Tohoku J Exp Med. 1956;64(3-4):301-3.

Clark AK, Haas KN, Sivamani RK. Edible Plants and Their Influence on the Gut Microbiome and Acne. Int J Mol Sci. 2017;18(5)

Craig WJ. Health-promoting properties of common herbs. Am J Clin Nutr. 1999;70(3 Suppl):491S-499S.

Crowell PL, Gould MN. Chemoprevention and therapy of cancer by d-limonene. Crit Rev Oncog. 1994;5(1):1-22.

Duthie SJ. Berry phytochemicals, genomic stability and cancer: evidence for chemoprotection at several stages in the carcinogenic process. Mol Nutr Food Res. 2007;51(6):665-74.

Fisk WA, Lev-tov HA, Sivamani RK. Botanical and phytochemical therapy of acne: a systematic review. Phytother Res. 2014;28(8):1137-52.

Lee CH, Wettasinghe M, Bolling BW, Ji LL, Parkin KL. Betalains, phase II enzyme-inducing components from red beetroot (Beta vulgaris L.) extracts. Nutr Cancer. 2005;53(1):91-103.

Osawa T. Nephroprotective and hepatoprotective effects of curcuminoids. Adv Exp Med Biol. 2007;595:407-23.

Van Lieshout EM, Posner GH, Woodard BT, Peters WH. Effects of the sulforaphane analog compound 30, indole-3-carbinol, D-limonene or relafen on glutathione S-transferases and glutathione peroxidase of the rat digestive tract. Biochim Biophys Acta. 1998;1379(3):325-36.

Yuan JM. Green tea and prevention of esophageal and lung cancers. Mol Nutr Food Res. 2011;55(6):886-904.

Chapter 4 – Be Kind to Your Gut

Jackson MA, Verdi S, Maxan ME, et al. Gut microbiota associations with common diseases and prescription medications in a population-based cohort. Nat Commun. 2018;9(1):2655.

Kim J, Ko Y, Park YK, Kim NI, Ha WK, Cho Y. Dietary effect of lactoferrin-enriched fermented milk on skin surface lipid and clinical improvement of acne vulgaris. Nutrition. 2010;26(9):902-9.

Kober MM, Bowe WP. The effect of probiotics on immune regulation, acne, and photoaging. Int J Womens Dermatol. 2015;1(2):85-89.

Kumar S, Mahajan BB, Kamra N. Future perspective of probiotics in dermatology: an old wine in new bottle. Dermatol Online J. 2014;20(9)

Logan AC. Dietary fat, fiber, and acne vulgaris. J Am Acad Dermatol. 2007;57(6):1092-3.

Maarouf M, Platto JF, Shi VY. The role of nutrition in inflammatory pilosebaceous disorders: Implication of the skin-gut axis. Australas J Dermatol. 2019;60(2):e90-e98.

Salem I, Ramser A, Isham N, Ghannoum MA. The Gut Microbiome as a Major Regulator of the Gut-Skin Axis. Front Microbiol. 2018;9:1459.

Vaughn AR, Notay M, Clark AK, Sivamani RK. Skin-gut axis: The relationship between intestinal bacteria and skin health. *World J Dermatol* 2017; 6(4): 52-58

Wolf R, Matz H, Orion E. Acne and diet. Clin Dermatol. 2004;22(5):387-93.

Chapter 5 – Protect Your Skin's Barrier

Ali SM, Yosipovitch G. Skin pH: from basic science to basic skin care. Acta Derm Venereol. 2013;93(3):261-7.

Bek-Thomsen M, Lomholt HB, Kilian M. Acne is not associated with yet-uncultured bacteria. J Clin Microbiol. 2008;46(10):3355-60.

Cao H, Yang G, Wang Y, et al. Complementary therapies for acne vulgaris. Cochrane Database Syst Rev. 2015;1:CD009436.

Chen YE, Tsao H. The skin microbiome: current perspectives and future challenges. J Am Acad Dermatol. 2013;69(1):143-55.

Chikakane K, Takahashi H. Measurement of skin pH and its significance in cutaneous diseases. Clin Dermatol. 1995;13(4):299-306.

Enshaieh S, Jooya A, Siadat AH, Iraji F. The efficacy of 5% topical tea tree oil gel in mild to moderate acne vulgaris: a randomized, double-blind placebo-controlled study. Indian J Dermatol Venereol Leprol. 2007;73(1):22-5.

Grice EA, Segre JA. The skin microbiome. Nat Rev Microbiol. 2011;9(4):244-53.

Prakash C, Bhargava P, Tiwari S, Majumdar B, Bhargava RK. Skin Surface pH in Acne Vulgaris: Insights from an Observational Study and Review of the Literature. J Clin Aesthet Dermatol. 2017;10(7):33-39.

Sohn E. Skin microbiota's community effort. Nature. 2018;563(7732):S91-S93.

Surber C, Humbert P, Abels C, Maibach H. The Acid Mantle: A Myth or an Essential Part of Skin Health?. Curr Probl Dermatol. 2018;54:1-10.

Zouboulis CC. Is acne vulgaris a genuine inflammatory disease?. Dermatology (Basel). 2001;203(4):277-9.

Chapter 6 – Treat Yourself Well

Bowe WP, Logan AC. Acne vulgaris, probiotics and the gut-brain-skin axis - back to the future?. Gut Pathog. 2011;3(1):1.

Bowe W, Patel NB, Logan AC. Acne vulgaris, probiotics and the gut-brain-skin axis: from anecdote to translational medicine. Benef Microbes. 2014;5(2):185-99.

Dalgard F, Gieler U, Holm JØ, Bjertness E, Hauser S. Self-esteem and body satisfaction among late adolescents with acne: results from a population survey. J Am Acad Dermatol. 2008;59(5):746-51.

Davern J, O'Donnell AT. Stigma predicts health-related quality of life impairment, psychological distress, and somatic symptoms in acne sufferers. PLoS ONE. 2018;13(9):e0205009.

Gorelick J, Daniels SR, Kawata AK, et al. Acne-Related Quality of Life Among Female Adults of Different Races/Ethnicities. J Dermatol Nurses Assoc. 2015;7(3):154-162.

Hamburg NM, Mcmackin CJ, Huang AL, et al. Physical inactivity rapidly induces insulin resistance and microvascular dysfunction in healthy volunteers. Arterioscler Thromb Vasc Biol. 2007;27(12):2650-6.

Lucey P. Sleep, leaky gut. Sci Trans Med. 2016;8(363):363

Misery L, Wolkenstein P, Amici JM, et al. Consequences of acne on stress, fatigue, sleep disorders and sexual activity: a population-based study. Acta Derm Venereol. 2015;95(4):485-8.

Romańska-Gocka K, Woźniak M, Kaczmarek-skamira E, Zegarska B. The possible role of diet in the pathogenesis of adult female acne. Postepy Dermatol Alergol. 2016;33(6):416-420.

Spencer EH, Ferdowsian HR, Barnard ND. Diet and acne: a review of the evidence. Int J Dermatol. 2009;48(4):339-47.

Chapter 7 – Supplement Wisely

Aikawa A, Mihara J, Tanida T, Tsukada S. The effects of glucuronic acid on acne vulgaris. Tohoku J Exp Med. 1956;64(3-4):301-3.

Bowe W, Patel NB, Logan AC. Acne vulgaris, probiotics and the gut-brain-skin axis: from anecdote to translational medicine. Benef Microbes. 2014;5(2):185-99.

Cervantes J, Eber AE, Perper M, Nascimento VM, Nouri K, Keri JE. The role of zinc in the treatment of acne: A review of the literature. Dermatol Ther. 2018;31(1)

Fouladi RF. Aqueous extract of dried fruit of Berberis vulgaris L. in acne vulgaris, a clinical trial. J Diet Suppl. 2012;9(4):253-61.

Jolliffe N, Rosenblum, LA, Sawhill J. The effects of pyridoxine (vitamin B6) on persistent adoslescent ance. J Investig Dermatol. 1942;5(3):143-148

Jung JY, Kwon HH, Hong JS, et al. Effect of dietary supplementation with omega-3 fatty acid and gamma-linolenic acid on acne vulgaris: a randomised, double-blind, controlled trial. Acta Derm Venereol. 2014;94(5):521-5.

Lim SK, Ha JM, Lee YH, et al. Comparison of Vitamin D Levels in Patients with and without Acne: A Case-Control Study Combined with a Randomized Controlled Trial. PLoS ONE. 2016;11(8):e0161162.

Pais P. Potency of a novel saw palmetto ethanol extract, SPET-085, for inhibition of 5alpha-reductase II. Adv Ther. 2010;27(8):555-63.

Rollman O, Vahlquist A. Vitamin A in skin and serum--studies of acne vulgaris, atopic dermatitis, ichthyosis vulgaris and lichen planus. Br J Dermatol. 1985;113(4):405-13.

Shokeen D. Influence of diet in acne vulgaris and atopic dermatitis. Cutis. 2016;98(3):E28-E29.

Siniavskiĭ IuA, Tsoĭ NO. [Influence of nutritional patterns on the severity of acne in young adults]. Vopr Pitan. 2014;83(1):41-7.

Snider BL, Dieteman DF. Letter: Pyridoxine therapy for premenstrual acne flare. Arch Dermatol. 1974;110(1):130-1.

Weber G, Adamczyk A, Freytag S. [Treatment of acne with a yeast preparation]. Fortschr Med. 1989;107(26):563-6.

ABOUT THE AUTHOR

Fiona Lawson is a former national magazine editor turned registered nutritional therapist. In her private practice and in her writing, she draws on the latest research to help people take charge of their health. With a special interest in skin, she has seen time and time again how a glowing complexion can transform self-esteem.

To read Fiona's blog, visit fionalawsonnutrition.com or follow her on Instagram @fionalawsonnutrition

Made in the USA
Monee, IL
10 April 2021

65386245R00056